Ultimate Self-Care is a must read for everyone. We are living in interesting times, where there are new devices, new stresses, and new illnesses, showing up every day on the planet. How do we navigate that? This book is an excellent guide, resource, and companion on your journey. You will learn why you may be experiencing what you are going through, and you will be taken through very practical techniques and tools that you can use from home, now. This book is incredibly put together with love, dedication, and a genuine caring for your own personal journey. *Ultimate Self-Care* is quite thorough and gives you more than just information. You will get tools, websites, and in-depth information to take you further. I highly recommend this book. Pick it up and form a group at your workplace. Imagine what could happen. If you start this book, you will never look back. Welcome to the first day of a new journey of transformation for you.

Dr. Divi Chandna, Intuitive Coach, Mind Body Spirit Center, www.drdivi.com

Ultimate Self-Care is a self-help book, and I love it. This book should be read by everyone. I don't think anyone could read it and not find something that resonates with them. It is the kind of book that you want to read again and start implementing some of the exercises. The author authentically shares her life experiences and philosophy. There is a great need for self-care, simply because our day-to-day life contains so much that is out of balance. Many of us suffer the stressors from work, family, and obligations, which rob us of our vitality. This book is a practical guide that starts with where you are. It asks you to take responsibility for implementing a strategy of self-care. The book is very well-written and smartly organized. It is a rare book amongst a growing pool of spiritual or new-age publications, which offers very practical guidance to people who are navigating their spiritual journey. Compassionately, Barbara Halcrow takes the reader step-by-step through every aspect of the deeper understanding of oneself. Her style is simple, flawless, and effortless, and the book is very well researched. It resonates with her own heartfelt and true experiences. I wish all workplaces could change their outlook and create balance by following the author's suggestion. The book is an overall winner to bring balance between work and relationship, with one's own self.

Bhavna Solecki, Founder/Director, Inner Evolution Center Ltd., Holistic Center for Pain and Stress Management, Vancouver, BC, Canada

Like the very definition of the term *ultimate* (incapable of further analysis; final; definitive), Barbara Halcrow's book *Ultimate Self-Care* is just that: absolutely definitive, comprehensive, and all-encompassing. It ranges in scope from a metaphysical, theological, and cosmic perspective on self-care, in relation to the core of our beloved planet, to the most practical pointers on how to practice self-care for oneself and others. Barbara is speaking about this topic from many levels: as a skilled counselor and social worker, a holistic practitioner, a spiritual visionary, and finally, as a human being, able to empathize with all manner of human experience. She has birthed this book from the very depths of her being, and the result is truly awesome.

Barbara's emphasis on the need for active and creative self-care is certainly in agreement with the premise of many doctors who integrate traditional and alternative medicine. So, Bernie Segal, in his book *Magic, Medicine, and Miracles*, spoke of working with exceptional cancer patients who were always active in their recovery, never merely passively surrendering to medical authority.

Deepak Chopra, in his latest book, speaks of the need for a healing lifestyle on every level, to counter the possible onset of any major disease. Barbara's book truly awakens this capacity for creative self-care and active recovery in anyone reading this book and following its precepts.

Dealing with constant stress and burnout is very much like being lost in a labyrinth. This book helps to provide the sacred thread that will lead us out of this maze. For anyone interested in self-care from any perspective, look no further. The answers have been given. What an extraordinary service Barbara has rendered.

Dr. Shirley Anne McMurtry, Vancouver, BC, Canada

Ultimate Self-Care reads well, is researched carefully, and covers a wide spectrum of spiritualties, philosophies, and psychology. When you interject your own experience and bring the suggestions and ideas closer to the reader, the goals become more attainable. Congratulations for a work well done, instructive, and useful. Many, many thanks.

Grazia Merler, Trento, Italy

If you have every wondered what "self-care" actually means, Barbara Halcrow has described what it is and why it is so important for us to take action to become more loving toward ourselves.

It's time to understand that self-care is not selfish. In fact, as Barbara points out, quite the opposite: without self-care first, we don't have a hope of being able to help anyone else on this planet or our mother earth.

Without knowing the truth of who we are and how and why we act in the world, we cannot possibly begin to learn to help and love ourselves or others.

As Barbara mentions, we are in an age of awakening, and as human beings, we move as energy rather than just matter. Barbara points out it is our vibrational frequency that we must become aware of; it affects our ability to communicate from our authentic selves. Embracing compassion, acceptance, and forgiveness increases our energy and brings us inner peace. I love what she says about energy, that "it can never be destroyed; it can only be changed or transmuted to another form," another vibration. This book is very detailed, with information on how each of our emotions carry certain frequencies and how that translates to our vibrational energy; this is important because we need to become aware that this is happening in our communications.

Barbara digs deep into explaining that without the awareness of taking action toward self-care, we risk living our lives from a place of stress and confusion.

She covers many topics in this book and gives you easy-to-follow steps to help you to become more self-aware and self-loving. Her steps help you to see how your thoughts affect your energy and how your energy is going out into the world.

Vibrational frequencies of emotions, although not a new topic, is going to become the next most talked-about form of healing. Eastern medicine has always known this, but only now is it broadening out into the Western world in a form that we can understand.

I highly recommend Barbara's book for anyone looking to understand what self-care actually looks and wants to know how to get there.

Chental Wilson
Author, *Can I Be Me without Losing You?* and *Pure Pilgrimage*

ULTIMATE SELF-CARE

A Holistic Guide For Strength And Balance In Changing Times

Barbara Halcrow, MSW

BALBOA.PRESS
A DIVISION OF HAY HOUSE

Copyright © 2019 Barbara Halcrow, MSW.

All rights reserved. No part of this book may be used or reproduced by any means, graphic, electronic, or mechanical, including photocopying, recording, taping or by any information storage retrieval system without the written permission of the author except in the case of brief quotations embodied in critical articles and reviews.

The information, ideas, and suggestions in this book are not intended as a substitute for professional advice. Before following any suggestions contained in this book, you should consult your personal physician or mental health professional. Neither the author nor the publisher shall be liable or responsible for any loss or damage allegedly arising as a consequence of your use or application of any information or suggestions in this book.

Balboa Press books may be ordered through booksellers or by contacting:

Balboa Press
A Division of Hay House
1663 Liberty Drive
Bloomington, IN 47403
www.balboapress.com
1 (877) 407-4847

Because of the dynamic nature of the Internet, any web addresses or links contained in this book may have changed since publication and may no longer be valid. The views expressed in this work are solely those of the author and do not necessarily reflect the views of the publisher, and the publisher hereby disclaims any responsibility for them.

The author of this book does not dispense medical advice or prescribe the use of any technique as a form of treatment for physical, emotional, or medical problems without the advice of a physician, either directly or indirectly. The intent of the author is only to offer information of a general nature to help you in your quest for emotional and spiritual well-being. In the event you use any of the information in this book for yourself, which is your constitutional right, the author and the publisher assume no responsibility for your actions.

Any people depicted in stock imagery provided by Getty Images are models, and such images are being used for illustrative purposes only.
Certain stock imagery © Getty Images.

Printed in Canada.

ISBN: 978-1-9822-3947-3 (sc)
ISBN: 978-1-9822-3948-0 (e)

Balboa Press rev. date: 12/20/2019

CONTENTS

Acknowledgments xvii
Introduction xix

Chapter 1: The Energy That We Are 1
    Have We Lived Before? 2
    The Body's Energy Systems 5
    Our Auras Are Extensions of Our
    Physical Bodies 5
    Seeing an Auric Field 7
    Auric Layers 9
    Chakra Centers 13
    Vibrational Medicine for Self-Care
    and Healing 18

Chapter 2: Our Body's Wisdom 23
    Cellular Knowledge 24
    Body Talk 28
    Made of Water 30
    Listening to Your Body's Messages 31
    An Exercise: Looking into the Mirror 32
    An Exercise: Checking in with Your Body ... 32
    Writing to Your Body 36
    Clarifying Our Natural Spiritual Senses 38
    Honoring Our Intuition 40
    Clairsentience 42
    Clairvoyance 43
    Claircognizance 44
    Managing Levels of Sensitivity 46

Chapter 3: Grounding, Clearing, and Raising Energy..51
   Meditating Is Easy..51
   Quick Start Meditation 53
   Heart of Compassion Meditation 54
   Easy Grounding Activities: Get Physical...... 56
   Are They Someone Else's or Mine? 57
   The Tree Root/Rose Clearing Visualization. 60
   Clearing by Smudging...................................61
   The Quick Overall Body Clearing Technique.. 62
   Mind Clearing Command............................ 63
   Chakra Clearing Using Musical Tones and Crystals 64
   Etheric Cords 66
   Cord Cutting 68
   Cord Cutting Exercise.................................. 69
   Clearing and Raising Home or Workspace Energy... 70
   Decluttering 71
   Smudging the Environment......................... 71
   Power in the Voice.. 72
   Drumming..74
   Using Color to Influence Energy 75

Chapter 4: Protecting Your Energy 83
   Your Surrounding Energy Field 83
   Exercise: The Egg and the Color of Violet.... 84
   Your Intention.. 86
   Invocations... 86
   The Importance of Our Personal Boundaries89

Know Yourself 94
Setting Boundaries 95
Saying No and Feeling Guilty 95
Assertiveness Exercise 96
Assertive Bill of Rights 98
Exercise: "Would I Allow My Inner
Child into This Situation?" 99

Chapter 5: Mindful Communications 101
The Conscious Mind 101
Default to the Negative 102
Media Watch 104
Communication in Stressful Situations 106
The Ease and Divisiveness of Gossip 107
Vibrational Levels of Emotions 109
Managing Changes 114
Self-Care Strategies during Change 117
Self-Care as Family Caregivers 120

Chapter 6: Building Our Resilience 123
Resilience 123
Nutrition in Self-Care 128
What Should I Eat? 129
Detoxification 133
Herbs and Spices 134
The Vibrational Color of Food 135
Blessing Our Food 137
Water 137
Water Quality 138
The Importance of Sleep 140

Insomnia 142
Suggestions for Improved Sleep 143
Physical Exercise..145

Chapter 7: Increasing Strength through Inner Doors 149
Every Feeling Counts 150
Listening to Your Heart's Wisdom..............152
Easy Heart Openings 154
Quiet Focus Within 155
Extending Love and Compassion 155
Gratitude..157
Music 158
Forgiveness 159
Forgiveness Exercise.....................................162
Staying Present in the Moment...................163
Managing Fear and Anxiety in the Moment 164
Cocreating What We Already Deserve 165
Three Guiding Questions 168
A Manifesting Process 170
Affirmations for Health and Wellness.........172
Synchronicity 173

Chapter 8: Self-Care Becomes Global Care...............177
The Earth Is an Intelligent Being................179
The Earth's Intelligence in Sacred Designs .182
What Earth Needs 188
Listening to the Indigenous Peoples............190

  How Individual Self-Care Affects
  Earth's Health 192
  Send Healing Thoughts to Earth 195
  Our Way through with Love 196

Chapter 9: Conclusion 201
Bibliography 205

Appendices 220
Appendix A 221
Appendix B 223
Appendix C 225
Appendix D 227
Appendix E 229

Index 235
About the Author 241

This writing is dedicated to anyone who feels the need for more self-nourishment, especially to those who give so much of themselves caring for others in their daily work or in their personal lives.

ACKNOWLEDGMENTS

I am grateful to many people who have encouraged me and taught me invaluable lessons throughout my personal and professional life.

In terms of my career path, I would like to offer my appreciation to the skilled women and men in their roles throughout the numerous areas of my work. Notably, Klinic Community Health Centre, Manitoba, and Vancouver Coastal Health, British Columbia, progressive health care organizations that offered me opportunities to expand my knowledge and give meaningful service to others.

Gratitude is also extended to my spirited and encouraging family members, Catherine Halcrow, Lindsay Barber, Betsy Parry-Greenwood, and Alison and Steeve Routhier. Special appreciation goes to Jean Halcrow, in spirit, who was singularly instrumental in kick-starting my writing.

Many thanks as well to Gisela Good, Brenda Whitehall, Carole Britton, Dr. Anne McMurtry, Anett Manering, and Audrey Clements (in spirit) for their insightful and consistent support.

To Doug Volz, a talented soul who gives us his heart-opening piano music that enriches me as I write.

Finally, my deepest gratitude to the eternal, guiding, and transformative energy of love that lies within each of us and gently calls us to trust in the voice and power of our own hearts.

INTRODUCTION

Are you feeling tired and stressed, with little time to care for yourself? Is your business or workplace going through continuous changes that leave you wondering if there is any downtime? Are you in the people-helping field or a caregiver to anyone, including a family member? Do you want to know if you can make more effective changes to improve some of your current self-care practices? This book is designed to give you additional ways through thoughtful, nontraditional means, to achieve better self-care and maintain greater health amid many of the changes and additional stresses that currently challenge us.

We seem to be in remarkable, changing, and uncertain times, with many kinds of systemic, cultural, socioeconomic, and global environmental challenges under way. Some changes are positive and add technological convenience to our daily tasks with innovative technological apps for online purchasing and all manner business development, as well as connecting us to the global market, the creation of smaller, more energy-efficient home appliances, and improved mass transportation systems, as only a few examples. There are new employment start-ups and technologies in some areas to advance human health as well as environmental health. While some forms of technological advances offer greater convenience, other changes are creating the opposite through fear, losses, trauma, and hardship.

Changes can result in sudden losses due to fiscal restraints or job obsoletion as a result of advancing automation; companies can relocate to other areas, leaving some communities in economic distress. We also continue to witness many countries undergoing significant political challenges and changes (e.g., Argentina, China and Hong Kong, the United Kingdom and Europe). In addition to dismantling of some previous political/economic unions, devastating wars also continue. Add in increased incidents of gun violence and terrorism in some areas of our world, to further injure far too many individuals. All these forms of strife and conflict can leave long-term traumatic impacts. Moreover, as we age, change our vocations, and experience various life events, changes in our own health can occur as well as the health of our family members, resulting in more of us adopting the role of personal caregiver to our disabled or elderly loved ones.

Overriding the aforementioned is the increasing magnitude and destructiveness of earth's climate changes, with major floods, fires, hurricanes, and earthquakes occurring worldwide; we're in a most remarkable and challenging time on this planet, a time where our levels of uncertainty, concern, and stress are increased. These global shifts are immense and can affect how we perceive our ability to go forward with concrete future plans. It also challenges all of us to take as good care of ourselves as possible in order to maintain our health, resilience, and sense of balance. Indeed, there is a lot going on, affecting each of us in various ways.

Focusing on our need for self-care is a loving and respectful thing to do. Giving proper nourishment to ourselves increases our vitality, self-esteem, and self-confidence. It not only improves our physical health; it also increases our mental and emotional clarity. Our self-care focus allows us to provide better support to others from a more energetic and balanced perspective. We ultimately can make better decisions about how much time and in what ways we can give to others. When we are better nourished, we can hear our own inner guiding voice more clearly.

Within my own life, I had many early challenges to overcome, beginning at a very young age. I grew up in a highly volatile, unstable home; both my parents had mental health and addictions issues and were unable to be fully present for me and my three siblings. I would often escape to the lakes and mountains near my home to find solitude and inner peace; I began to experience a deep and abiding spiritual connection to the natural world. This strong connection contributed to me being able to hear my own inner voice, which helped guide me spiritually in the following years to find the additional help and direction I needed. Over time, with the assistance of many supportive, loving healers and others, I was able to move through many emotional challenges with more ease. It was from the grace and wisdom acquired from those difficult yet transformative years of my life that I am able to see more clearly that all of our life experiences have meaning and purpose, even if we don't fully understand what they all mean at the moment. I was able to acknowledge later on that my parents were actually two of my greatest teachers in my life's journey, and for that learning, I am grateful.

Ultimate Self-Care: A Holistic Guide for Strength and Balance in Changing Times is a unique holistic guidebook that combines many areas of personal and professional experience and study. For over twenty-five years, I have practiced as a counselor, energy healer, and social worker, and I held leadership roles across the continuum of health care. These areas include working with people challenged by addictions, mental health issues, abuse, physical disabilities, and many kinds of traumatic life losses. In all of these experiences, I have remained aware of how our energy or spiritual essence of each of us is interconnected with our physical, mental, and emotional selves. Therefore, the focus in this writing has also included this recognition of our human need to address our spiritual needs, whatever that may mean to each of us.

During my career in social work and teaching, I have always tried to be vigilant about my own health. I have also been concerned about the health and wellness of clients, colleagues, friends, and family. In this regard, I have personally experienced the struggle many people have to care for ourselves in practical, balanced ways, ways that take into account the challenges of our work and our need to embrace many changes, while we also deal with the range of our personal life experiences, the joys as well as sudden losses that we find in our journeys.

Throughout this book, I reference many people who are involved in various aspects of the spiritual realm or energy work around the world; we are in an age of conscious awakening, an age of rediscovering what our ancient ancestors knew: that we are human beings of moving energy rather than just inert matter, and as such, we are actually capable of doing more for ourselves in shaping our lives for the better.

We can experience some of this awakening unfolding as we can participate in numerous experiential mind and body healing forums and retreats around the world. We can also view much more information available to us via new publications, programs on various cable channels, and internet sources. This information is revealing historical and current information that had not been shared to such an extent. The variety of investigative commentaries and in-person interviews from scientists, archeologists, health experts, metaphysicians, and academic scholars provide education across the broad spectrum of mind/body/spirit subjects; learning opportunities continue to expand exponentially.

Ultimate Self-Care: A Holistic Guide for Strength and Balance in Changing Times encourages a more holistic approach to our self-care. We can take an active role in participating in improving our wellness and our happiness, especially when we are experiencing extra stress. Self-care from a holistic approach more fully embraces the mind/body/spiritual aspects of who we are. These areas, therefore, cover not only our physical needs, but also what builds strength and resiliency for the breadth of who we are as human beings.

When we include a focus on caring for the fullness of our humanness, we can change our lives more effectively, knowing that as we attend to one area, it will also help support other areas because the mind/body/emotional/spiritual systems are integrated. Therefore, our diet in the foods we eat and the beverages we drink affects not only our physical body, but our emotional, cognitive, and mental health states, leading to our overall sense of well-being. Additionally, what we choose to read, view, and believe in can affect our physical energy as well.

This emphasis on self-care is not about becoming selfish or self-serving; it is about appreciating all aspects of what we truly need to create wellness, strength, and balance in our lives. We can support ourselves more effectively when we understand how to work with all our energy systems.

When we know more about our own body's intelligent systems, we can rejuvenate ourselves by clearing, raising, and protecting our energy. We can become more aware in recognizing situations that have the potential to adversely lower our energy, and in doing so, we take preventative steps to maintain our balance and help avoid ill health.

As we care for ourselves and become more fine-tuned with the full range of our natural spiritual senses, we also evolve our appreciation of how we are beautifully made, holistically constructed, and sacredly interwoven in our connection to all the life that surrounds us.

This guidebook looks at many areas of self-care as we attend to our daily routines, at home or at work. Self-care can be a series of small steps that can be managed even in high-stress situations; each step or activity that feels right and doable becomes important in moving in the direction of wellness.

There is so much information that is coming forward and changing daily that this book's approach as a guidebook will work well. For as much as I have benefitted in my own health by writing this guidebook, I sincerely believe you will also benefit by using its many practical suggestions in the exercises, strategies, and resource links provided.

This book will provide you with information on understanding the interrelationship of your mind/body/spirit connection and the ways you can use this powerful interconnection to lovingly raise up your vibration to optimize your physical and emotional health and achieve a deeper sense of inner peace and spiritual freedom. Understanding this interrelationship of your holistic energy systems gives your greater insight into more effective ways of advancing your self-care practices. This book includes the following information:

- How to have a positive impact on your body's functioning by communicating directly with it and receiving its information
- How to use easy ways to clear, raise, and protect your energy at home and at work
- How mindful communications can uplift and strengthen you and those around you
- How to encourage your heart to be more open to allow an increased flow of compassion and acceptance of yourself and others
- How your improved self-care practices will help raise the vibrational frequencies within you, around you and how it can extend to positively impact the health of the earth

Each of us is meant to be here during this remarkable time of change in our history. The importance of truly knowing who we are as holistic beings and what we are capable of doing to improve the health of our lives and of this planet cannot be understated, for we are at our own crossroads to make important choices, choices that will ripple across and touch many other souls on their paths.

Even during increasing societal and cultural changes and challenges that bring us personal uncertainty, losses, and confusion, we can still seek ways to stay balanced, healthy, and resilient. We can do this by choosing to open to the deeper knowledge that lies within us and is being made available to us. We can practice nourishing ourselves with more loving-kindness, compassion, and appreciation, the same kind of kindness and tender nourishment that many of us offer to others in our lives.

My hope is that this book will provide supportive reminders, practical information, and other forms of guidance that resonate with you and encourage your self-care in whatever ways feel right for you.

Appendix E offers a self-assessment tool to aid in creating your own self-care plan. You might want to review this section before beginning your reading, as it may make the book's contents more relevant to you.

CHAPTER 1

THE ENERGY THAT WE ARE

If you want to find the secrets of the universe, think in terms of energy, frequency, and vibration.

—Nikola Tesla

We are far more than what we appear to be. Physically, mentally, emotionally, and spiritually, we are intelligent energy systems that are interconnected with all of nature. Every cell contains the pattern of our existence (Lipton 2008, 162).

This is not new information, but not until recently, with the advancement of technology, did our scientific community fully embrace what ancient cultures instinctively knew about our relationship with the cosmos—that everything within us and connected to us on this planet and throughout the universe is composed of vibrating atoms and, as such, is eternally in motion (Maclean 2006, 15).

Obviously, we cannot see this energy vibrating with the naked eye, but we can feel it and often sense it. Even seemingly lifeless objects such as rocks vibrate, but they do so at such a low level, we might erroneously assume they are dead and have no energetic life force. We now know this is not the case.

We also witness material breakdowns, decay, and changes in the material world constantly transpiring around us, as all earth forms energetically shift and transform or transmute in the reappearing processes of life and death. We have greater understanding of energetic changes from the physics that tells us energy is never created or destroyed; it can only be changed or transmuted to another form (Moskowitz 2014).

This scientific information is powerful in its overall implications. it implies that as physical energy forms, we are also transmutable and infinite. Although our physical bodies will die in terms of our chemical and electrical systems that shut down and decay, we still debate the existence and afterlife of the energy of human consciousness, soul, or spirit.

Have We Lived Before?

There is accumulating evidence through accounts of individuals' otherworldly experiences that may guide us toward understanding the human soul as a conscious energy that endures beyond our earthbound existence. Dyer and Garnes' (2015) *Memories of Heaven: Children's Astounding Recollections of the Time before They Came to Earth* is a compelling read of unsolicited stories of past-life experiences, specifically of what they felt and saw while in the dimension of heaven, as reported by their parents.

Another book, *Life before Life: A Scientific Investigation of Children's Memories of Previous Lives,* is scientifically researched and presents fascinating interviews with children who recalled detailed memories of their previous lives, including precise locations of where they lived, how they died, and information about their previous family members and their livelihoods. Upon investigation, these reports were verifiable, giving rise to the serious premise that our consciousness may continue beyond the brain's death (Tucker and Stevenson 2008).

There are also documented stories of adults who have gone through near-death experiences. Through those spiritual journeys, they have returned to provide us with profound life-altering stories. One extraordinary and medically verified report is from Dr. George G. Ritchie (2007), who was pronounced dead for nine minutes and returned with life-changing information about his journey. Not only did he travel around the medical room to view his own deceased body; he also consciously transferred his spirit to another part of the country. Lastly, he reported that he traveled to another dimension, where he received information from those in spirit form before finally reentering his body.

You are not a drop in the ocean. You are the entire ocean in a drop.
—Rumi

Researchers in varying fields continue to investigate the nature of our energetic existence. One organization looking at multiple levels of inquiry is the Institute of Noetic Sciences (IONS), founded in 1973 by Apollo 14 astronaut Edgar Mitchell (https://noetic.org/about/).

After Mitchell returned from space after a life-altering event, he established IONS to investigate and advance the understanding of the spectrum of his experience. The institute uses tools and techniques from all existing sciences that involve neuroscience, psychophysiology, cognitive and personality psychology, computer engineering, and physics to comprehensively study the nature of intuition, consciousness, distant healing, mind-matter interactions, and individuals' transformative experiences (McNeil 2006, 8).

As he traveled back to earth, Mitchell's powerful epiphany left him transformed in his understanding of the nature of human consciousness in connection to the universe around him. He later relayed the following statement of this event in an interview with Dr. Barbara McNeil, his colleague at IONS:

> My understanding of the distinct separateness and relative independence of movement of those cosmic bodies was shattered. I was overwhelmed with the sensation of physically and mentally extending out into the cosmos. The restraints and boundaries of flesh and bone fell away (Ibid.).

He went on to say that this same experience was more like a "savikalpa samadhi" moment—a moment whereby "an individual recognizes the separateness of all things, yet understands that the separateness is but an illusion" (Ibid.).

From Mitchell's impetus and the many researchers who have signed on in the past years, IONS explored the nature and expansiveness of human consciousness and how it interacts with the world; the organization's notable members have been published in distinguished academic scientific publications.

The Body's Energy Systems

There is much more documented scientific evidence concerning the intelligence of the body and the mind-body connection; as we will continue to note throughout these pages, it becomes easier to appreciate that in our human energetic construct, our bodies seem to have their own intelligent and complex energy systems that work collaboratively and synergistically to function and create optimum health. One of the best things we can do to support our overall health is to understand the areas of ourselves that we normally do not physically see but can definitely experience.

As vibrational beings, we continuously shift and expand our energy in conjunction with our sense of wellness. Our overall energy is influenced by our thoughts, attitudes, beliefs, and feelings, and they, in turn, come full circle to impact our physical health. These interwoven energy systems create an electromagnetic charge that naturally extends outward and can be experienced by people, animals, and plants. All living matter has an energy field, and the energy that extends outward is called our auras.

Our Auras Are Extensions of Our Physical Bodies

When two people meet, within seconds, they have an impression and can assess the kind of energetic vibe that is being given off. We assess if we are comfortable with this person or not and determine what mood or frame of mind that person might be in. This vibration can be felt subtly at times, or there might be a greater presence about a person who gives a stronger aura.

Some people have strong personalities, and their auras can be more intense and even extend out further from their bodies. Sometimes, without seeing or hearing them, we can feel people's auras when they come near us.

The auric field is made up of seven layers, which I will discuss in detail later in this chapter. Each layer is connected to different parts of us and holds a different frequency. This means each layer receives information that comes from our physical selves—from our organs, blood, bones, hair, skin, and every other cell that makes up the human body. All of these parts are constantly sending and receiving information. These electrical and chemical intercommunications are reflected out into each of the corresponding layers in this auric field.

Dr. Carolyn Myss calls our surrounding auric field "a highly sensitive perceptual system" and agrees that all matter has an energy field because "everything is alive and pulsates with energy and all this energy contains information" (1996, 33).

We are holistic beings, completely interconnected in that our physical functioning affects our emotions, minds, and spirits—like an outer mood ring, if you will. Auric layers change their frequencies and colors as we shift and change our emotions, mental states, and temperaments.

For example, as we make an emotional shift, our auras will mirror a higher vibration if we are feeling happy and well; they will pulsate at a lower vibration if we are depressed or angry. Altogether, our auric fields reflect our overall health, our personalities, our temperaments, our beliefs, our mental activities, and our emotional states. They reflect everything going on within us, and this is where our biography becomes our biology.

Seeing an Auric Field

People can be trained to read and interpret auric fields; they can also see where an imbalance or disease is present or at risk of occurring. Unless we have learned to develop our natural inner sight or are medical intuitives or clairvoyants, we generally do not physically see this energetic extension of our physical bodies, but we can certainly feel it. If we could all consciously see one other's electromagnetic auric fields, we would see that they measure about three to nine feet around us, depending on the person's health and wellness.

People who work with healing the energies of the body, such as Reiki practitioners, develop their intuitive abilities in sensing the auric field; many can actually see it. Most experienced energy healers can pick up the energies emanating from the auric layers in the field and interpret the body's energetic data being expressed. They will be able to sense the areas of strength or depletion in the layers of the auric field and offer ways the client's body can be strengthened and healed.

Although not a common experience for me during the course of my personal and professional practices, I have occasionally seen aspects and colors of people's auric fields. These experiences began to occur more often when I became involved in spiritual/energy studies, as well as in situations during my regular practice as a social worker.

In one experience, I clearly saw the entire auric field surrounding one of my spiritual teachers become a soft emerald green. It was so large and visible, it appeared like a translucent blanket that covered her aura, her entire energy field. This occurred as she was teaching me an intense heart-centered meditation, and we were calling in maximum healing energy to be involved in the meditation. It was a powerful moment for me to witness. The same energy eventually filled the room for several minutes; it felt exceedingly peaceful, loving, and calm.

In another situation, I was in a professional meeting and witnessed the subtle white light energy of a colleague flow across the table to touch the energy field of another practitioner she was speaking to. It was immediately clear to me that this colleague's words had a greater impact in that moment because her energy carried her mindful words, which were also infused with the compassion from her heart.

This combination of the heart informing the mind is where wisdom lives. I have had other instances where I have seen white light completely cover a person's auric field. This light tells me the person is in a very open state and is receiving a higher vibration of energy coming from a very loving source.

Ultimate Self-Care

Auric Layers

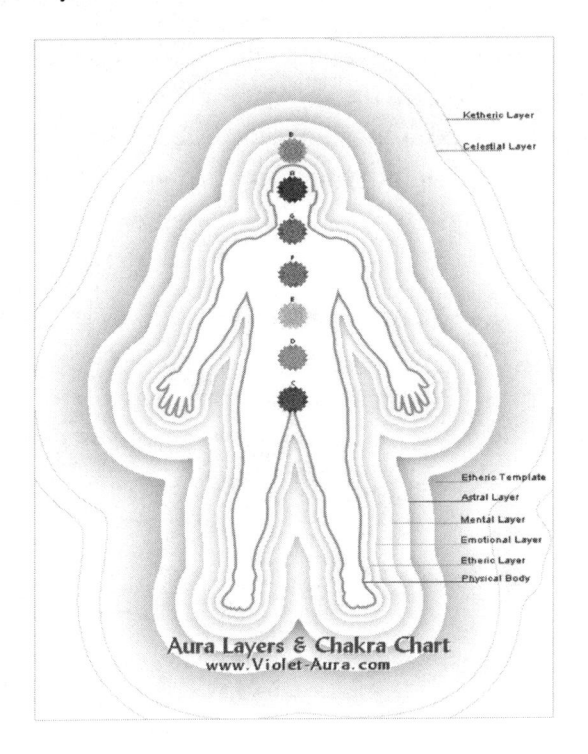

(Permission to print: www.violet.aura.com)

This auric diagram gives a visual idea of our outer auric field of energy and what each layer means from the first layer, closest to the body, to the outermost seventh layer.

To understand the auric body apart from the descriptions in this text of the referenced auric layers and colors, they are easily found on websites simply by entering "chakra colors."

First Layer (Etheric Layer)

This layer (red in color) is closest to the physical body; it is really a subtle form of the physical body. The energies of this layer are awakened through practices like yoga, tai chi, and qi gong, or by simply paying close attention to the energies, especially the breath.

Second Layer (Emotional Layer)

The emotional body (orange in color) is connected to our feelings, and it can change colors like a rainbow, according to the changing feelings of the person.

Third Layer (Mental Layer)

The mental body (yellow in color) holds our thoughts and mental processes. The primary color associated with this layer is yellow and can be seen more around the upper body with the head and shoulders.

Fourth Layer (Astral Layer)

The astral layer (green in color) acts as a bridge to the spiritual plane. The colors of the rainbow are present within this field of energy but can be seen as mostly a pink hue if the person is involved in loving, healing work. This level is also the emotional level that connects to the heart chakra and emotional body.

Fifth Layer (Etheric Template Layer)

The etheric template layer (blue in color) can be seen by those gifted with clairvoyance as a deep blue and is closely related to the throat chakra.

Sixth Layer (Celestial Layer)

The celestial body (indigo blue in color) is related to the sixth chakra or third eye (or "mind's eye" of inner knowing or perception), and it is associated with spiritual enlightenment, unconditional love for humankind, intuition, and higher degrees of feelings and thoughts.

Seventh Layer (Ketheric/Causal Layer)

The seventh ketheric or causal layer (violet in color) is the body that contains all other bodies within it. This layer is associated with serenity and the universal or divine mind, and it contains all the information of the soul's journey through all of time (what is referred to as the akashic record).

As you can see, the auric field involves our psychological mind, our emotional nature, our physical body, and our spiritual selves. From a systems perspective, what affects one part of our selves affects all the other parts. As vibrational beings, we inherently strive for an energetic balance or equilibrium. Being balanced is what we actually feel when we are in a place of calm and peace. Given the stresses of the world, we know that balance can be difficult to achieve and maintain.

Now we will look at the master whirling engines of our human system, our chakras: specific and highly sensitive energy vortexes strategically located within our body to disseminate information around the body and through to our auric field.

(For various examples of the colors noted in our auras, please see www.violet-aura.com.)

Chakra Centers

Chakras are energy-awareness centers. They are the revolving doors of creativity and communication between spirit and the world.
—Michael J. Tamura

In the ancient Eastern language known as Sanskrit, *chakra* means "the wheel." Chakras are considered to be the major energy centers of spiritual power in the body. They do not fluctuate in their location. They remain stationary in our body and distribute life energies throughout our body and also connect through to our auric field.

In Indian, Ayurvedic, or life-knowledge medicine, illnesses in the body are related to chakra imbalances, blockages, or misalignments. When our chakras are not spinning properly in a clockwise direction, it can cause discomfort that might be manifest as a sense being out of sync, minor tension, an inability to fully focus or concentrate, a result of our natural spiritual connection to life and our life force, or chi, being slowed down.

This lack of chi in our vibrational system can be felt in our physical energies being slow and lethargic, a sense of depression, and even disconnection with ourselves and others. We can also experience a lack of cognitive clarity, feel unable to be happy, or lack self-esteem and self-confidence. This kind of situation can place anyone in a far more vulnerable place to turn to addictive substances to boost their low energies in more artificial ways.

The chakras spin in a clockwise motion (away from the base of the spine toward the head crown). Each of our chakras is prescribed a dominant color that has a similar vibration as the chakra itself. Specific crystals, musical tones, and even fragrances have vibrational measures that match each of the seven chakras. Each chakra has a connection to an organ as well as to one of the endocrine glands (Wills 1993). The specific colors assigned do not mean that they are always actually seen as such. Many healers strongly intuit the chakras instead of seeing them in their color hues.

Each chakra has a distinct purpose, and there are effective ways of healing these energy centers to allow them to move properly after they are interrupted by an emotional, physical, or mental event, causing an imbalance or illness. Overall, when we exhibit a physical illness, it most often will first have been experienced as a spiritual or emotional disturbance, an unresolved hurt, injury, or trauma. This disturbance will not only slow down any of the chakras, but its impact will also make its way through to our outer body's auric energy field.

The seven main chakras shown in the next image are referenced most often in literature in terms of how they connect to our other energy systems; they can reflect imbalances that can potentially lead to ill health or disease.

Ultimate Self-Care

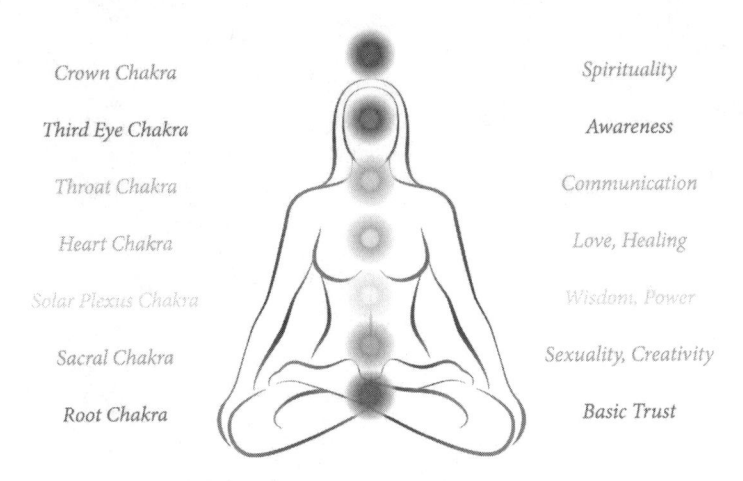

Crown Chakra — Spirituality
Third Eye Chakra — Awareness
Throat Chakra — Communication
Heart Chakra — Love, Healing
Solar Plexus Chakra — Wisdom, Power
Sacral Chakra — Sexuality, Creativity
Root Chakra — Basic Trust

(Photo: Peter Hermes Furian. Permission to reprint.)
https://www.freeart.com/artist/peterhermesfurian/

First (Root) Chakra is red in color, and the focus is with energies that feel vital and active.
Physical: adrenal glands for the flight-or-fight response, immune system, the base of our spine, rectum, legs, feet.
Imbalances: lethargy, sluggish, emotionally or physically inflamed, angry, depressed, unable to focus.

Second (Sacral) Chakra is orange in color and involves our gut or intuitive feelings, sensuality, inner wisdom, curiosity, joyfulness, appropriate boundaries with parents.
Physical: colon, bladder and gallbladder, pelvis, sexual organs, hip, appendix, and adrenal glands.
Imbalances: mood swings, excessively strong emotions, disconnection from core self.

Third (Solar Plexus) Chakra is yellow in color. Its primary focus is the sense of "I" in our use of the intellect, knowledge, strength of will, self-assertion, and personal power.

Physical: digestive system, liver, pancreas, middle back muscles.

Imbalances: diabetes, chronic fatigue, hypertension, sarcasm, blaming and confused thinking.

Fourth (Heart) Chakra is green in color and is centrally located; it acts as a critical link between the first three chakras and the fourth to the seventh. This chakra's focus is on healing, wholeness, a sense of something greater than ourselves, love, transformation, serenity, insight, relationship connectedness, compassion, and empathy.

Psychological: a shut-down or blocked heart chakra will become critical, judgmental, jealous, cold, too self-sacrificing.

Physical: heart, circulatory system, cardiac nerves, lungs, thymus, breasts, chest area, arms.

Imbalances: heart disease, lungs, immune system, upper body pain.

Fifth (Throat) Chakra is blue in color and is concerned with communication, oration, voice resonance, truth telling, deeper listening, peace, and calm.

Physical: throat, thyroid, neck, parathyroid, mouth, teeth, and cervical spine.

Imbalances: all areas mentioned; communication issues, verbal domination, confusing messages, falsehoods, and blocked creativity.

Sixth (Third Eye) Chakra is in indigo color and allows for heightened sensitivity, insights, integration between the observable and the unseen worlds, imagination, visualization, strength in mental clarity, and focus. The pineal gland is widely known as the seat of the soul and is the size of a small pea, located centrally in the brain. It deals with the brain's functions, pituitary and other glands, head, eyes, and nose.

Imbalance: memory loss, lack of perception and objectivity, delusion, obsession, and emotional imbalance.

Seventh (Crown) Chakra is violet in color and is our welcoming, open connection to the divine, infinite spirit, and cosmic oneness in spiritual consciousness. It is ultimately about our ability to become energetically balanced and to attain unity and reconciliation within us and with all other forms of life, composing varying degrees of female and male energies (yin and yang). This reconciliation of energies produces a complete sense of love, peace, and harmony. In keeping this chakra open, we remain curious and alive in life's learning.

Physically: involves our brain, cerebral cortex, skeletal system, and skull.

Imbalance: brain tumor, autism, crown headaches, ego's domination in any area, greed, emotional dissociation, apathy, depression, and feeling ungrounded.

Whether we are able to see, sense, or simply just appreciate the fact that we have a highly intelligent energy system embodied within each of us, it can support us in our self-care when we feel out of balance. When we have felt out of balance, many of us have sought energy treatments or vibrational medicine, without naming it in this way, to help us to rebalance. I have continuously received Reiki healing and other forms of vibrational medicine to rebalance my chakra system and heal other stress-related issues when they occur.

Vibrational Medicine for Self-Care and Healing

The natural healing force within us is the greatest force in getting well.
—Hippocrates, Father of Medicine

Energy is also medicine. Many people have sought vibrational medicine or some form of vibrational treatment in their lives. Treatments using sounds and specific musical tones, such as crystal bowls, chimes, or the human voice for chanting, as well as the use of nature's own remedies found in herbs and flower essences, are just a few examples in a long list of vibrational medicine healing techniques. (Other examples are listed at the end of this chapter.) In recognizing ourselves as beings composed of energy, Gerber (2001) states, "Vibrational medicine uses specialized forms of energy to positively affect those energetic systems that may be out of balance due to disease states." The essential goal of vibrational medicine is to use forms of energy to move, unblock, or rebalance our own body's energy to prevent illness or to eradicate disease.

Within our more traditional medical systems, practitioners like physiotherapists rely on vibrational energy in the form of ultrasound waves to provide an energy balm for sore muscles and often combine it with transcutaneous electrical nerve stimulation for pain reduction.

Ultrasound waves are used to decrease the healing time for soft tissue inflammation in the post-acute phase by increasing the blood flow to the injured area, as well as increasing the production of more collagen to positively affect the formation of scar tissue (Virtual Sports Injury Clinic 2016)

Vibrational medicine is also used to surgically remove malignant organs or tissue; for example, laser light can cut or destroy a cancerous tumor. Lasers are also used in eye surgery (e.g., cataract removal), and most recently, vibrational energy treatments have been adopted within the cosmetic industry for hair removal (electrolysis). For people interested in weight reduction, private companies are now using radio waves to heat up fat cells under the skin, causing their demise, whereby the body then flushes them away. The list grows.

Practiced on a regular basis, our daily self-care can affect all five of our senses. Some of these supportive practices are easy and can help you to calm down or get energized, such as incorporating more whole green foods containing more energy, spending time in nature, listening to soothing musical tones, spending time with loving animals, or practicing simple meditation. There are a variety of other examples that will be offered in the chapters ahead.

Vibrational energy healing techniques that Western society has recently become more familiar with have long been considered as the first order of care in other cultures. They are itemized below, and some methods are described in more detail in the chapters to follow.

Reiki

The Japanese practice of Reiki originated as a touch therapy, using specific hand positions held above or on the body. Reiki works in support of all body systems and is particularly powerful in addressing chakra vortexes that are out of balance and re-establishing the energy flow, which in turn assists in all aspects of our healing.

Acupuncture

Acupuncture, thought to be three thousand years old, originated in China. This modality stimulates the body's own healing processes by using very fine needles gently placed into the skin on selected points on the body.

Reflexology

Reflexology assists in the body's own healing processes and is used by Western and Eastern cultures. It is a touch therapy that acts to prevent illness or respond to physical or emotional distress. Reflexology utilizes specific reflex points found in hands, feet, and ears that have corresponding nerve pathways or meridians connecting to all parts of the body.

Breathwork

There are many forms of vibrational healing therapies that involve breathwork. Specific patterns of breathing exercises are incorporated into different practices to enhance the participants' complete holistic health. Yoga and tai chi also use breathwork to improve self-awareness and address mental and emotional issues.

Homeopathy

Homeopathic remedies are actually diluted doses of natural substances that are effectively used to cure the same symptoms they can cause. This method of treatment stimulates the body's own healing mechanisms.

Flower Essence

Flowers and plants each have a specific energetic frequency, and as such, flower essence preparations encapsulate the frequency that can assist in specific healing of the individual. Additionally, these preparations enhances the positive consciousness of the person in their connection with nature.

Healing Sound Therapies

Sound therapy or sound healing involves the human voice, as in chants, drumming, Tibetan singing bowls, tuning forks, and gongs, all for the purpose of vibrationally stimulating the natural healing energy of the body. Instead of traditional surgery using cutting procedures, surgeons in London have already used sound waves deep in the brain to help relieve a patient of his Parkinson's tremors. There will be more of these kinds of treatments to come.

Barbara Halcrow, MSW

Colored Light

Each color has a different wavelength and therefore a different frequency. Color is used in many ways to enhance our emotional, physical, and mental energies. The effective use of color to help in our care and healing is discussed at length in chapter 3.

Crystals and Gemstones

Crystals and gemstones have found their way back into our consciousness to advance healing and health practices, though they have been utilized since ancient times. Crystals hold higher vibrational frequencies than other stones and are also important conduits of energy, as we see with the use of them in our various technologies. The use of crystals and stones is discussed further in chapter 3.

To sum up, it makes sense as vibrational beings that we are open to consider the full range of proven vibrational medicine and treatment methods that can align with our body's intelligent network of cells, energy centers, and fields to balance, heal, and maintain our health. I believe we can easily see that the future of medical treatments and healing methods will use sound and light waves with greater success, resulting in less intrusion for patients.

CHAPTER 2

OUR BODY'S WISDOM

Everything you need to know is within you. Listen. Feel. Trust the body's wisdom.
—Dan Millman

As we now appreciate that all words, beliefs, and actions we hold true about ourselves are continuously being reflected in our body's experience, we can become actualized in our approach to health. It is important to try to be conscious about what we are actually saying, not only to ourselves in how we feel about who we are, but also how we feel specifically about our own bodies.

We know our bodies are intelligent, interconnected energy systems. Our cells are also intelligent and aware of us in ways we may not have realized. Our bodies have wisdom and are indeed listening, taking in everything and everyone we encounter, including all experienced environmental stimuli, visual images, and even those images created from within our own imaginations.

According to Candice Pert, science has proven that each and every cell in the body carries the full memory of every single thing we have ever thought and experienced as well as the compaction of unresolved issues still festering away, as they wait to be released (Pert 2008–2016). Pert found through complex biomolecular experiments that the body and mind are involved in a constant, responsive, and dynamic information exchange in which cellular memory was evidenced (Pert 1997, 144).

Barbara Hoberman Levine says our body is like an emotional barometer. She posits that discomfort within our bodies can, at minimum, initially point to an area of emotional distress. Our bodies will never lie to us. That is why in order to find answers, we can also look within and fine-tune it, listening to how our bodies are feeling (Levine 1991, 69–78).

Our bodies are always responding when we are able to pay attention to the signals. For example, if we are in an acute or prolonged state of stress of any kind, our bodies will begin to signal that stressful discord with aches, pains, nervous energy, and sleep disruptions; later on, we may experience a more pronounced set of responses and symptoms to tell us to take immediate action to resolve our imbalance and alleviate a potential illness or disease.

Our spiritual, emotional, intellectual, and physical realms are in constant intercommunications, showing us the immense interweaving of the intelligence that we are. It also allows us to know that the more holistically aware we are, the more we can consciously influence positive change within ourselves and in our bodies, regardless of our genetic makeup.

Cellular Knowledge

Science is recognizing that genes do not control every characteristic of our lives; they are not the equivalent of the cell's brain. Recently, the biological science of epigenetics

Ultimate Self-Care

has shown us that cellular behavior is most profoundly influenced and even altered (without changing the genetic code) by our conscious beliefs and our environment.

This cellular intelligence is not held within the nucleus, as one might assume, but rather in the membrane surrounding the cell, which receives signals directly from our environment. Environmental signals include environmental issues and biological, psychosocial, and cultural influences and patterns in our lives, expressed in our overall lifestyles.

Dr. Bruce Lipton (2008), renowned for his scientific research in the area of epigenetics, supports earlier civilizations' long-held spiritual and esoteric worldviews that all matter has, at its most basic elemental core, a consciousness, intelligence, or spirit that underlies its behavior.

The wisdom of the body is very real. This more recent scientific view tells us that rather than being controlled or even victimized by what has been passed down to us in our genetic code, we can make choices in our environment and take greater mastery over our genes.

Lipton argues that changes in our minds, beliefs and visions of our world, leads to chemical changes in our blood, which does not change our genetic construct but it ultimately influences how our genes behave (Ibid., xxvii). [1] This means that we can influence the way our genes express themselves by being aware of what we truly believe in, the kinds of environments we live in, the impact of who we are surrounded by, how we nourish ourselves in mind/body/spirit; these all have influence on how our genes will

---

[1] Bruce Lipton also has a video series referencing his work. (https://www.youtube.com/watch?v=G4T0LzU_rv0)

respond. The conscious intelligence of our cellular bodies and their interrelationship with our spiritual, emotional, and psychological selves can be more clearly recognized.

With this recognition, it is far easier to appreciate that there are entire cellular communities within us, consciously performing specific jobs and responding continuously to the impact of our thoughts, words, sounds, as well as ingested food, air, water, the influence of others, and even the fabric and colors we wear. Our bodies are fully responsive to all our senses and to all the energies we are involved with (Ibid., 100–102).

Because we are energetic, vibrational beings, our understanding of the brilliance of our bodies' intelligence and capacities holds the potential for more miraculous breakthroughs in the healing arts and medical fields. Bartlett (2007) says that some of the information coming forward via epigenetics and matrix energetics, as examples, is not really new but rather ancient spiritual and shamanic insights and techniques being brought into our present-day consciousness (x).

Cellular communities with a purpose: This is a micro definition of who most of us are as complete whole beings, naturally part of our own collection of social and functional networks and communities, contributing to our sense of purpose and happiness. Sondra Barrett, a biochemist and immunologist from California, examines how each of our cells experiences its own intelligent purpose and reason to be a part of the particular community in which it thrives (Barrett 2013, 73–84)

This understanding that cells are conscious and aware of their own purpose can be extrapolated on a much larger scale that purports that cells in all living organisms on this planet are in fact sentient, with the ability to feel, perceive, and experience their existence subjectively. Ergo, all of life is truly energetically alive.

If we consider this vital awareness of life being so dynamically alive in whatever energetic form, it gives rise to many issues, including how we can consciously send positive messages to our bodies to assist ourselves in every area possible. Dangeli (2007–2017) claims there is a direct form of bio-communication between you and your own body. It means for example, that we can be even more conscientious in preparing our bodies for surgery, recovery, and self-care afterwards. The clearer the messages, in even simple conversation with our bodies, in terms of what is going to happen to any of our body parts, if they need to be altered or removed, and countless other considerations, can help alleviate some of the stress and potential trauma our bodies can experience.

This information is not so different in terms of how we would give vital information to a person who is about to undergo a medical procedure, whereby clients are encouraged to learn as much as possible about health care recommendations in order to more fully participate in their own healing. In my experience, people who work more collaboratively with their health care practitioners and prepare well, usually experience a better recovery. Therefore, verbally communicating with our body as a means of supporting our own health is not an absurd thing to do;

rather, it is a very real, effective, and loving way to offer more caring for ourselves. In this next section, I'll share an example of some of the ways I prepared my body prior to surgery.

Body Talk

At age forty-five, I had to undergo hip surgery due to severe osteoarthritis. By that time, I had already learned a few things as a therapist and social worker about doing visualizations and speaking to my body. I therefore decided, before this surgery, to fully prepare myself, in all ways possible. I researched the procedure and spoke to my body about it. I explained exactly what was to take place. I asked my body to prepare to say goodbye to the part of my hip that was worn out. I thanked my hip for taking me as far as it did throughout my life and asked my body to accept the new cellular material that was going in surgically. It was a conversation with myself, similar to planning with a family to accept a newly adopted member with loving support.

In the course of that preparatory time, I developed my own pre-surgery and post-surgery visualizations, along with healing colors that I could use afterwards to ensure I would heal as fully as possible. These visualizations involved imagining and feeling, in advance of the surgery, that I was fully relaxed, organized, and prepared for my surgery, as were the nurses, surgeons, and anesthetist. I sent prayers in advance to assist the surgeons and all medical staff, so they'd be guided and well-supported in their work. I sent loving white light into the surgery room a day ahead, as I have experienced sending in love and white light into countless other situations that might be potentially challenging. Over time, I am sure it has helped contribute to a more relaxed and peaceful flow of energies between people.

After surgery, I visualized soothing, healing colors of green and pink for my body. I also spoke to my body with love and gratitude for its remarkable ability to cope and to heal. I continue to talk to my body whenever I feel the need to inquire about an organ or muscle and to encourage any needed healing.

A fascinating report, "Scientists Prove DNA Can Be Reprogrammed by Words and Frequencies" (Fosar and Bludorf 2011), states that we can create positive physical effects (through influencing our DNA) by using our own language with simple words and sentences. Fosar and Bludorf report on a Russian molecular biologist, Pjotr Garjajev, who examined the large amount of "junk" DNA that scientists seemed to have almost no information on; he and his colleagues found that this extra DNA is not only responsible for our physical functioning, but it also acts to store data and plays a role in communications within our body.

They found this information by exploring the vibrational levels and responses of our DNA. They put specific frequency patterns onto a laser ray, and when modulated, they saw that could influence DNA frequency, thereby influencing the genetic information of the DNA. This experiment validated their understanding that the basic structure of DNA and of language are actually the same. This particular finding was one of many aspects of a range of newer findings regarding our DNA. In taking far more into account than can be explained in this brief reference, Garjajev and his colleagues said that our human DNA is really own biological internet and is superior to a computerized instrument, in that it can be influenced by words and frequencies.

"This finally and scientifically explains why affirmations, autogenous training, hypnosis and the like can have such strong effects on humans and their bodies. It is entirely normal and natural for our DNA to react to language" (Ibid., par. 5).

Although few of us will ever be involved in scientific DNA cellular research, we can appreciate the immense wonder of our incredible capacity to recover and heal. We can do this by paying attention to what we are thinking, what our emotional states are, and how our bodies are feeling, in terms of where our pain or stress resides. We can also heal more effectively from illness and surgery and assist in our total mind/body self-care by simply speaking lovingly and supportively to our body and tuning in to listen for its messages to us.

Made of Water

Thinking and speaking lovingly to our bodies will become more conscious when we also recognize that we are primarily composed of water. Our water composition has implications. Dr. Masaru Emoto, throughout his book, *The Hidden Messages in Water* (2009), described experiments in which he froze water droplets and then analyzed their crystalline structure. Prior to freezing, each separate water droplet was offered a loving word or, conversely, a negative word or phrase.

Later, when examined microscopically, the droplets that had loving words imparted to them exhibited beautifully formed crystalline designs, like snowflakes. The droplets exposed to negative words showed chaotic and disorganized structures. The water cells were obviously affected according to the energy of words given to them.

As simple as this experiment sounds, it is also worth paying attention to when we know we are composed of 92 percent water. It tells us of the importance of thinking and speaking with kindness, caring, and love to our bodies, the very kind of words we would give to a dear friend.

Listening to Your Body's Messages

By accepting that our bodies really are listening to us, we can be as understanding and compassionate about ourselves as possible. Many of us feel that we have some measure of physical imperfection we want to change, and our body feels the thoughts of rejection we send it. We can judge ourselves as not perfect or see ourselves as not good enough or feel inadequate, as compared to the glossy images of attractive, supposedly perfect-looking men and women staring at us from the magazines in grocery aisles, on TV, or from ads throughout social media. It then becomes far too easy to judge and assess ourselves: We are too fat, we are too thin, we have low muscle mass, our hair is thin, our nose is too big; the list becomes endless. The misperceptions and societal distortions presented to us have contributed to creating a sense of distance from our own genuine humanness, our true remarkableness, and our need to love ourselves exactly as we are. It has overall contributed to a sense of grievous separation from our body, which has ultimately taken us away from the truth of our body's wisdom and our connection to the divine.

The following series of exercises will help deepen your connection to your body and your body's true need to be loved, accepted, and nurtured, as you would want to care for someone you really love.

An Exercise: Looking into the Mirror

As a simple suggestion and initial practice on a daily basis, try this when you look into a mirror:

See your own reflection without judgment, condemnation, or rejection. Thank your body and tell it, "I accept you, and I love you," for everything it has given to you. As you have already travelled some distance in this world in your physical vehicle, your body is really an amazing and invaluable friend – even if you feel it has confused you - or more likely you've not understood its messages. When you give your body simple words of acceptance and caring that it deserves to hear, it will receive your positive energy on a cellular level. The more you practice giving truly loving nourishment to your body in word and action, the better it can respond.

An Exercise: Checking in with Your Body

Another simple exercise you can do is to check in with your body when you can. It takes a couple of minutes, at most. This check-in allows your body to give you direct

Ultimate Self-Care

information. Keep your expectations low in terms of receiving immediate inner verbal messages or images, if you have never tried to communicate with your body before. You might only get subtle impressions or words as answers, but all we really need is a word or a physical sense to tell us what we intuitively already know.

Scan Your Body

- First, simply sit comfortably in your chair. Take three deep breaths into your abdomen. For each breath, count to four as you slowly inhale, then hold your breath to the count of four, then exhale slowly to the count of eight.
- Mentally and emotionally, tune inward and scan your body, beginning from the top of your head and go down your back and arms; check out your abdomen and your legs to your feet.

Notice where you are feeling tense or have aches and pains; you may already suspect why you hold tension in various areas. You may know that your chair isn't ergonomically supportive to your body or that certain lights are too bright or not bright enough, thereby putting strain on your eyes, or that you feel the stress of a high work load or deadlines, or there may be specific physical duties that are becoming too challenging. Perhaps there's too much chatter or noise around you to allow proper focus on your tasks.

You might notice these areas of tension and stress:

- Does your head ache? Do your eyes water? Is your jaw clenched? Is your brow furrowed?
- Where are your shoulders? Are they moving up toward your ears?
- Are your hands clenched?
- Is your stomach knotted?
- How are your legs and feet feeling?
- Is there an area in your body that holds the most tension, or do you experience your whole body as being constricted?

If you feel like you are holding tension, make a note of it and consider taking a step to support releasing this tension as soon as possible, as tension accumulated over time tends to worsen.

If you do this body scan at work, consider walking around your work area, go outside for a break, or do some additional deep breathing for a few minutes to more calming. If at home, soak in an Epson salt bath, arrange for a massage or another appropriate complimentary health practitioner, or see a counselor, if need be.

Information that your body gives you is vital; we may at times dismiss or suppress our feelings, but our bodies will not lie to us. Our feelings will always be revealed, as the body will eventually tell us what is truly going on.

In your scan you may want to notice if some of these physical tensions come about only in certain situations or specific environments; if you weren't aware already, that will give you more information about what's contributing to your emotional stress or irritation.

Ultimate Self-Care

Ask Your Body What It Needs

To find out more answers, approach your body with genuine concern and compassion. Tune inward and simply ask your body, "What do you need?"

- Physically, is your body hungry or thirsty? This may sound simple, but we can be confused if we are hungry or thirsty. A lack of good routine nourishment or hydration will in itself create an energy drain, followed by other mental and emotional symptoms of depletion.
- As you focus on your body, ask, "What do I truly feel, and what do I need?" Be aware that an immediate answer of "Sugar, please," in the form of baked goods, for example, may not be the wisest choice, but that kind of message will tell you that you are likely wanting a quick energy boost (or, conversely, your body really needs to rest and not be pushed harder). An alternative to a strong sugar hit might be lemon in water, fresh fruit, some nuts, or a piece of cheese. I anticipate an energy drain in midday and usually have the alternatives I have just mentioned, and they are also good on-the-go snacks.
- Do you need to move? You might have thoughts or feelings that tell you your body needs to get up, walk around, or get outside, perhaps to be a few minutes in nature, near trees, or something else you might already be aware of but may not have made time for. Sometimes we are inclined, or

feel forced, to push our body beyond its capacity due to personal demands and expectations or work responsibilities and pressures.
- Thank your body for communicating its messages. Your thoughtfulness in terms of listening carefully and properly attending and nourishing your body can take time, especially when we feel overly stressed with insufficient downtime.

Writing to Your Body

Another exercise that can allow you to go deeper in your communications with your body is to simply write down a question to your body, a specific body part, or organ to receive an answer as to its functioning. What is it trying to tell you? Why is it in discomfort? Is it holding in any sadness? People have written to their lungs, kidneys, legs, and other parts of their bodies, and have received significant information.

You may get inner impressions, emotional insights, or feelings that can be emotionally painful events from the past that may still be affecting you and are manifesting physically. Aside from dialoguing directly with your body, writing or journaling is an effective way to allow information to come forward from your body.

Prior to my own surgery discussed earlier, as I tend to journal regularly, I wrote to my right hip when it was in pain. I simply wrote the following:

Ultimate Self-Care

"Dear Right Hip,

"Why are you in pain? What has happened, and how can I help support your healing?" I waited for any kind of inner feeling and response to come. To facilitate a message back, I wrote, "Dear Barbara". I then waited, and a message came: "I feel a lot of sadness and grief that I need to express. I also need you to listen to me when I am tired and not push me or demand I work so hard." I felt this message to be true for me.

You may not get any information at the first go of this kind of writing. You may get a feeling, a one-word answer, or like me, a full-on reply. However, as I wrote, I did feel sadness well up in me. I had already been involved in doing other emotional healing work on various life circumstances. At that time, I was able to more fully comprehend that my body was carrying my memories, my experiences over this lifetime.

What arose in my body's fuller response to me was the sudden death of my brother from an overseas car accident, when I was twenty-one years old. This death was a traumatic loss, and after so many years, residual grief was still being held in my body, although I believed I had emotionally resolved his passing.

Besides the hip joint, I also discovered there was more sadness being held in my upper chest that I could feel on occasion. I have come to appreciate that our unresolved feelings can be tucked away in multiple places, until there is a point when it accumulates and becomes an overload of stress for our body, and our immune system will begin to suffer. Often when we are able to release one memory of sadness, for example, other losses may be dislodged, giving rise to more feelings of hurt and sadness that have waited their turn to be recognized and cleared.

It seems clear that our body holds wisdom through our cellular memories and also through its immediate responses to people, places, and things that come onto our path on a daily basis. Our body remains our truth barometer, or ultimate lie detector; it will always tell us in some way what is going on in any situation, negatively or positively.

In any moment, you can experience your body's messages by consciously focusing and tuning into your body, specifically your solar plexus, as your gut-sense barometer, to feel your way through any situation you feel unsure about.

I worked extensively as a counselor with abused women who still lived at home in domestic violence circumstances; one of the important pieces of developing a protection plan was to have them listen to their intuition or their body's gut sense in order to feel out if their body felt "safe" or "not safe" at certain times at home. This practice is effective in honoring the instinctive senses we all have to feel, to know, what may be potentially hazardous to us.

Before I became more tuned in to my body's ways of conveying information to me, I relied on other areas where I experienced information coming to me. We will look at some of our natural intuitive or spiritual senses next.

Clarifying Our Natural Spiritual Senses

"People have always understood intuitively that mind and body are not separable. Modernity has brought with it an unfortunate dissociation, a split between what we know with our whole being and what our thinking mind accepts as truth. Of these two kinds of knowledge the latter, narrower, kind most often wins out to our loss" (Mate 2012, xi).

Within the richness of our humanness, we all have natural spiritual gifts with which we arrive. We may have suppressed, denied, or acculturated to regard our sensory gifts as part of our own so-called crazy imaginations. Some people believe our extrasensory natures to be a negative aspect of who we are that needs to be expunged. Thankfully, our natural human senses are being accepted and expressed more openly to give all of us a chance for more personal exploration and development.

If we want to increase our intuition, we need only start paying more attention to it and follow through with those inner guiding nudges that we often call our gut sense. It will naturally increase our intuition. Those nudges will become stronger and clearer, giving you greater insights as you validate them. I would always recommend journaling your experiences because it can be invaluable to be able to review and to connect up the experiences we are having; sometimes, we discover patterns or themes to explore further.

Those who have more developed intuition may also have other sensory gifts available to them when receiving extraordinary information. This information can come from within from our inner or higher selves or, as some would believe, our guides, the angelic realm, or even deceased loved ones spiritually existing in another dimension on the other side.

Where these messages come from is up to us to discern. Even people who have not had experiences in these areas can receive these kinds of messages or information at various times and remember them as curious, minor events. Or perhaps they may have been profound moments that touched our hearts, opened our minds, and offered a rich glimpse into another realm available to us.

My strong belief based on my own experiences is that the more we value our spiritual senses and fully understand them, the more information we can bring in to guide our own lives. I have benefited enormously when I decided to listen to my body, my intuition, and my other senses as described in the instances below. This kind of honoring, listening, and following creates more strength and confidence in us as we learn to trust ourselves more deeply.

Honoring Our Intuition

In essence, intuition is also referred to as our higher instinct and is part of our survival senses. It also means knowing without really knowing, sensing something might happen in a certain way, or feeling that we need to take a certain action, without being able to articulate exactly how or why that knowing exists. When we have ignored our gut sense, our instinctual intuition, we might have heard ourselves saying, "I knew I should have done that. Why didn't I listen?" We've often regretted it.

I recall a time when I was ready to leave work at the end of a Friday. I was tired, but I decided to extend myself by making one last phone call to an ill client to see if they received the health information I'd mailed them. It wasn't really necessary, but I didn't want to feel I'd left any dangling ends before I left for the weekend. I didn't listen to my own needs when feeling mentally and physically tired. I also

Ultimate Self-Care

dismissed my nudging intuition which told me to just to go home.

I made the short call and proceeded home in my car. As I crossed a bridge (now being about ten minutes behind my normal schedule), a bus in front of me suddenly snapped its trolley line, and the line veered straight for my car. I ducked as it hit the top corner of my car, barely missing the windshield, then it bounced over to strike the car in the next lane beside me, only to rebound back again and smash into my back passenger window, obliterating it. Fortunately, no one was hurt, but the lesson was notable for me, to not only pay attention to my mental and physical signals when I'm tired, but also to listen when intuitive warnings are given to me.

There are other times when I want to make a decision about a situation, but I am hampered by this sense of knowing something is really off. I cannot put my finger on it, and I seem stuck. It's not necessarily from being afraid of making the wrong decision. It usually means that the timing of the decision is off, in terms of other events behind the scenes being lined up in my life, or there is a lack of information to allow me to fully decide what to do. When this kind of scenario happens, it's best to wait, to remain patient, to trust the process for both the timing and additional information to be settled; you will feel it in your body, you will intuit it, and you will make a clearer decision.

Along with our intuition, we have other natural spiritual gifts. You may resonate to any of the following:

Barbara Halcrow, MSW

Clairaudience

Clairaudience means clear hearing. It is our ability to receive words and sounds, internally or externally, that may not part of the regular sensory realm. Sometimes, it is hearing specific sounds or voices or music that is not discernable to the normal ear. For example, when I was a new motor vehicle driver, I was driving alone and about to turn left onto another street. Just before I made the turn, a very loud voice shouted on my right side, "Don't turn!" It really startled me and made me hesitate for just a second, only to see a speeding car narrowly miss me, as it suddenly appeared from nowhere and turned right into my path. We would have had a terrible head-on collision if I'd continued with the turn.

A more common occurrence for internal information arriving for me is when I am meditating or simply concentrating on an issue and want to have an answer, I just ask the question, and I often will "hear" an immediate answer with exact wording. I believe this form of clairaudience is more familiar to people than is appreciated. The best thing to do in terms of strengthening this ability is to simply ask the question, listen, and write down the very first answer that comes to you.

Clairsentience

Clairsentience is a clear sense where one is able to discern at a distance another's feelings, with no plausible explanation as to how it can be known. This extrasensory ability can occur when we have a strong, distinct feeling fall over us without explanation, feelings we can also experience on a physical level. This kind of experience has been well documented over time; it often comes up between parent and child or loved ones who are at a distance and an illness or injury has occurred. Some people are able to do this at a distance, without ever being familiar with the person at a distance. Many people who have these experiences are also very empathic; they sense other's feelings easily and tend to absorb them. However, I am a strong empath but am not advanced to the extent that I can instantly or clearly discern other's feelings, unless I choose to meditate or focus on tuning in to them.

Clairvoyance

Clairvoyance is clear seeing or vision, where one is able to gain information about a person or situation at a distance through visual telepathy. This is also referred to simply as extrasensory perception. One of the most famous clairvoyants in our history was Edgar Cayce (1877–1945), who exhibited profound abilities while in deep sleep and trance states. His work continues to be studied to this day. Although I have received only random visual hits of others I might tune into or am asked about, the most profound forms of clairvoyance have come through my own premonitory dreams. Since I was a young child, I have had significant dreams, and throughout the years, I've recognized that my dream life is a great source of information about what is going on more deeply within me, as well as what is going on with others, including what may be pending in the future.

For example, when I was a social worker in the Yukon, I had a dream that depicted two teenaged sisters I was

Barbara Halcrow, MSW

working with in a foster home. They wanted to visit their father in another town, far away. My dream, unfortunately, told me that if they travelled by car, there would be an accident, and they would not survive. I was distressed at this dream and asked my supervisor whether to share this information as a warning in my professional capacity as their social worker. The supervisor felt it was worth mentioning this information, in case they could make alternative travel plans. I let the girls and foster mother know of my dream and said that perhaps it was a sign to be heeded. I explained that I had these kinds of dreams from time to time. They decided to travel by car, after all. Unfortunately, the dream materialized; there was a fatal car crash, and one of the girls died immediately, while the other was hospitalized for a lengthy period of time. As one can imagine, especially in any smaller community, it was an emotionally heartbreaking time for all involved.

To increase your dream recall, keep a dream journal by your bedside; as soon as you awaken, write down whatever dream fragments come to you. In time, you'll slowly begin to recall your dreams more fully, and you will discover a world of themes, messages, warnings, and an increase in your own creative potential being given from within.

Claircognizance

Claircognizance is clear knowing that is more than just intuition. It is a very developed sense of knowingness that transcends time and can allow a person to access information about situations in the past, present, or future. It can involve predictions, premonitions, and flashes of immediate insights

Ultimate Self-Care

that cannot be backed up with any concrete explanation. This is a spiritual gift that I have found within myself that has risen up since my early days, quietly but significantly. The information arises as needed and as one is ready to receive it. As meditation and relaxation enhance all spiritual insights, they also enhance claircognizance.

A simple example was while I was relaxing with a friend years ago, I suddenly knew in a moment that my mother was going to pass away in two weeks. My mother lived at a distance, and there was no evidence, given her relative youthfulness, to suggest her death would be imminent, but she died from a sudden heart attack exactly two weeks to the day after I said it. The knowing, as I can best describe it, is a clear whole-being or mind/body/spirit kind of experience and feels irrefutable when the sensory information comes through me. Other examples have occurred over time, but this insight was one of the most startling for me.

If you wonder how to develop this sense of claircognizance or knowingness, I can say, as with the other areas mentioned above, it is important to keep a journal; validate your hunches, feelings, and senses. You might be doubtful about your experiences, but choose not to doubt; choose to explore your senses, instead. We all have these spiritual or energy senses as part of us. In fact, I will venture to suggest they are not really gifts per se. We have grown away from our natural ability to recognize and use all our senses, after centuries of conditioned separation from our spiritual selves, for fear of being thought of as odd or even crazy. Throughout human history, intuitives and healers have often been put to death for exhibiting their spiritual senses.

Barbara Halcrow, MSW

I constantly rely on the breadth of my intuitive senses, and I will always strive to listen to them in order to further strengthen them. Overall, I can say with absolute certainty that when we give all our senses the attention and validation they deserve, we will strengthen our capacity to provide ourselves with more accurate information. When we are inquisitive about our extraordinary yet wholly natural senses and tune in to them more closely and consistently, decisions will become easier, and our lives can run more smoothly. [2]

Managing Levels of Sensitivity

Each of us is uniquely, expressively different; people who are curious acquire more learning and validation about their own personality aspects, communication styles, preferences, and sensory sensitivities.

There are countless formal and informal tests and questionnaires available that range from assessing superficial aspects to assessments that are far more in-depth and comprehensive. Popular personality assessments are easily accessible online but are not always reliable. Online questionnaires can be found that purport to test for various sensitivities such as empathy but only offer a cursory analysis of those qualities. There are also some excellent books, articles, and online resources available that can be helpful and contribute to good emotional self-care methods. One of the first books regarding sensitivity levels, and still an excellent read for personal self-exploration, is *The Highly*

---

[2] There are formal and informal ways to develop our natural spiritual senses. See appendix A for additional resources.

Sensitive Person: How to Thrive when the World Overwhelms You (Aron 1996).

People who experience the world more sensitively might be more developed or gifted in these "clair" areas; they can also react in ways that can be confusing to themselves and others, thus contributing to unfortunate misunderstandings. A need for withdrawal or retreat, feeling nervousness or agitated, with additional immune system issues, allergies, and other associated symptoms can be a few signs of extra sensitivities that are being overloaded. They feel the need to detach from someone, a situation, or an environment, until they are able to rejuvenate.

It's to our benefit to know how to recognize our areas of sensitivities and determine if there are areas we need to manage, protect, or heal. It is also well worth exploring, if there are additional traumatic experiences adding to any of our responses or triggered reactions.

Sensitive, intuitive, empathic people have the ability to quickly feel and absorb others' emotions. These people are found in all walks of life and occupations, as one would guess, and those of us who experience our senses acutely need to manage our intuitive, empathic natures well in stressful environments or in roles that are less geared to be feeling focused. You'll usually find intuitive empaths gravitate more toward the healing arts or helping occupations that allow for easier self-expression and acceptance.

Highly sensitive people can take more time to reconcile their desire to seek advancement into leadership roles, for example. The reason is that they can perceive, rightly or not, that there could be an increase in degrees of stress and subsequent feelings of becoming overwhelmed when facing situations with more wear and tear to the nervous system.

Additionally, even if we consider the impact of social, psychological, cultural, and gender factors, sensitive people may experience lower levels of ego strength, because they focus on what they need to learn rather than appreciating wisdom they have already acquired. This trait can be displayed in shyness, self-deprecation, and self-consciousness. Ergo, they may feel they are less equipped to go forward when, in fact, their insights and inner wisdom offerings are what some organizations may really need.

An interesting conundrum is that occupations like health care, education, social services, and direct caregiving—where sensitive intuitives, healers, and empathic people are liable to gravitate—are often cited as some of the highest stress positions; all levels of staff are vulnerable to feeling overworked, overwhelmed, and burned out. I can attest to this issue in my own life's work as an intuitive empath and a social worker; it's been challenging to seek higher roles while providing myself good self-care amid ongoing, accumulative stress.

Markowitz (2013, chapter 3) argues that many empathic people will tend to mask, manage, or cope with their sensitive natures, vis-à-vis the barrage of ongoing and cumulative levels of workplace stress by consuming alcohol or other drugs, including over-the-counter medications, to deal with increased anxiety, stress-related nervous disorders, chronic fatigue, and sleeplessness.

From my own perspective, most people are actually a lot more emotionally sensitive than they may be aware of. This reticence can sometimes be a result of a cultural, gender, or

Ultimate Self-Care

work-setting issue, with men more often feeling withheld than women to recognize or reveal their intuitive, empathic, and sensitive natures.

Overall, managing our emotional sensitivities, or some of the higher acute senses, remains an important focus for self-care. It's helpful if this self-care involves some knowledge about clearing and grounding our energies, as well as asserting our boundaries and other supportive protection measures within our work or home environments. Some of these strategies are addressed in the next two chapters.

CHAPTER 3

GROUNDING, CLEARING, AND RAISING ENERGY

If every eight-year-old in the world is taught meditation, we will eliminate violence from the world within one generation.
—Dalai Lama, 2012

Meditating Is Easy

To meditate is to focus, clear the mind, and bring oneself into a more relaxed state while sitting or lying down comfortably. Meditation is an excellent way to help relieve stress. It uses the breath in a regulated manner to bring in calmness and assist the mind to step out of its constant chatter. The benefits of practicing simple daily meditation have been well documented. These benefits include calming the mind and grounding the nervous system, reducing stress, creating inner connections with oneself, shifting perceptions to allow for increased creative thoughts, expanding a loving connection with all life, and the list goes on.

Practicing meditation is actually very easy. It's about focusing and being present. For a long time, I didn't warm up to the notion of meditation until I realized I was already doing informal meditations, when I went into deeper conscious mind states when I wrote, painted, gave in-depth counselling sessions, and even quietly tuned into music.

Later on, when I began to take more formal meditations through my spiritual training courses, I found the restful clearing benefits became greatly enhanced. Once you decide on a time and place to practice meditation, you can easily develop it as a habit. The truth is, you can meditate as you need to, indoors or outdoors.

There are different kinds of meditations; one that is well known is called Transcendental Meditation, founded by the Indian guru Maharishi Mahesh Yogi. It incorporates mantras and chanting, and uses various energetic vibrations in sounds that can assist in opening us to different levels of consciousness. To develop the habit of being mindfully present, meditating in the morning is usually a good place to start.

There are many simple meditations that can be practiced daily; all you need is a quiet space for from five to twenty minutes, whatever works as a beginning point, as well as for your schedule. Some people like to build up their meditation time and start at two minutes, then five minutes, and on from there. In essence, meditation is about being focused and present while also focusing on your breath. [3]

---

[3] For more resources for accessing guiding mediations, see appendix B.

Quick Start Meditation

I've used this simple form of meditation over the years, at various times of the day or evening, with good results. It helps you become calmer and more relaxed.

Sit or lie down wherever you are that is comfortable and allows you to focus.

Focus completely on your breath. Take three deep breaths: breath in and hold your breath for about four seconds and let go slowing for about four seconds. This breathing in and out will begin to immediately calm you. Then shut your eyes and continue to closely focus on your breath. Again, with eyes closed, take three more deep breaths as before, as you slowly exhale. As you focus on your breath, your mind may continue chattering, trying to tell you all the things you should be doing in that moment. Choose to ignore the chatter and keep solely focused on your breath, in and out, in and out. Focus on your breathing for as long as you can, even if only for ten seconds. It will still be very helpful to turn your attention inward and become quieter inside.

If you want to try another easy breath technique that uses a different rhythm, I suggest the video on Dr. Andrew Weil's 4-7-8 Breath Technique.[4] He has a brief video offering a good example of a breathing technique that is simple and effective.

---

[4] Andrew Weil (http://www.drweil.com/videos-features/videos/the-4-7-8breath-health-benefits-demonstration/).

Barbara Halcrow, MSW

Heart of Compassion Meditation

For me, in addition to focusing on my breath, I have also tuned into my heart chakra as the most powerful energy center from which to begin. Our hearts are powerful and can guide us in how we can compassionately and clearly move through this world to bring peace from within and then send that compassion out to others.

Some people like to light a white candle for a spiritual focus in meditation, but it is not necessary. If you want to keep your eyes open, then looking at a candle is an excellent focus point. If you are not in a place to use a candle, just choose another focus that has some kind of meaning, reflecting love or nature.

1. You can sit on a chair or sofa, sit cross-legged on the floor, or fully lie down. If you choose to sit down, ensure your spine is straight with your feet on the floor and head positioned looking straight ahead for a good energy flow. Just be comfortable.
2. Place your hands palm up on your lap or in another mudra position. There are many positions to hold your hands and fingers for different meditations, and they each hold meaning in their correspondence to various organs.

For this meditation, you can use the Shuni Mudra. This simple body connection with the fingers allows for more focus in your meditation, which can help quiet the mind; in that way, energy can flow more smoothly throughout the body.

Ultimate Self-Care

As well as the intention for the meditation and the healing benefits that go with each one, there are many good websites to give you an idea of the sacred meaning of the mudras.[5]

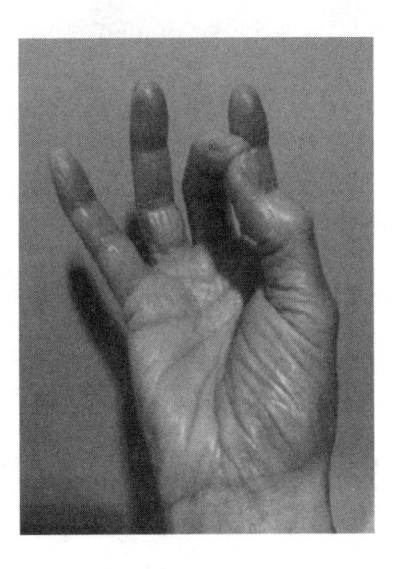

Shuni Mudra: middle finger and thumb tips connect in touch and assists to help one remain present. (http://www.harisingh.com/newsMudras.htm)

1. **Focus on your breath** and inhale a deep, slow breath (count from 1 to 4) in through your nose and then out through your mouth (count from 1 to 4). Do this exercise three times.
2. **Focus on your heart**. Think of your heart having a beautiful, slightly closed pink rose within it. Think of the animals and people you love. Send them your

---

[5] www.harisingh.com/newsMudras.htm

love, and see your love for them being returned back to you, into your heart.

As you breathe, continue to focus on this rose, and see it slowly open up its petals. As it opens, it also opens you to receive more love, kindness, and compassion. Ask for love, kindness, and compassion for yourself and for all living beings.

3. **See the loving pink energy** from this rose expanding to include your whole heart, then further expanding to fill your whole body. Envision this pink, loving light energy now filling your room, home, or work setting, and then expanding to fill the whole building.

Continue to visualize this healing pink light filling the entire neighborhood, then your state, then the country you live in, until you are able to visualize this energy completely surrounding the earth.

The energy of extending these loving thoughts for yourself and toward others is real. It is an extremely positive thing to do and makes a difference in ways you may never be aware of, but extending love, kindness, and compassion is soothing and ultimately healing. Others do receive it, and as energy flows, it will be returned to you, again and again.

Easy Grounding Activities: Get Physical

Our physical bodies contain earthly elements, and the earth's gravity helps us become connected with our physicality. Below are a few examples to put you in caring

Ultimate Self-Care

touch with your body, when you need to relax or use your body. Animals can offer emotional, unconditional love to directly nourish your spiritual nature, which ultimately helps our minds and bodies. These examples help in overall grounding our energies:

- have a body massage
- sit in water with Epsom salts or simply take a shower
- walk in nature
- garden
- work with clay, sand, or dirt
- dance, run, walk vigorously
- eat root vegetables
- house clean and declutter
- go to sleep earlier for a longer rest
- be with loving animals
- roll a tennis ball under your feet to help relax various muscles
- get a foot massage

Clearing Energy
Are They Someone Else's or Mine?

Thoughts as sparks of energy can fly faster than a blink of an eye between one person and another. Watch what happens in any meeting or with anyone you're with, and you may experience knowing exactly what is going to be said next. This inner happens because we can sense the patterns of speech being used in our specialized work arenas, and other times we are simply tuning in and receiving distinctive thoughts being sent out by those around us. You can try a quick experiment by repeating in your mind a distinct thought and sending it out into the room to see who picks it up.

This connection we have with each other through our thoughts and feelings can happen at any distance. Thoughts, being energy, have no trouble travelling through time and space in a millisecond. For example, when a major tragic event occurs anywhere on the planet and large numbers of lives have been lost, with ongoing trauma being experienced, we might not yet be aware of what has happened across the globe, but we will feel a collective sense of those energies to varying degrees.

We are also aware of those times when we suddenly think of someone out of the blue, and they call us, or we connect with them and are told with surprise, "You have been on my mind," or "I was just thinking of you." You can call this phenomenon a form of energy transference or telepathy, since we are all telepathic, like every other animal in the world.

At times, we can suddenly feel drained, depressed, anxious, and unmotivated. Sometimes, we know exactly why we feel this way, but other times, it's not clear. These feelings can happen frequently when we have been in stressful situations and around others who are experiencing difficult circumstances, even if they don't tell us about them. There are times I have felt a sudden flush of various energies by simply travelling on public transit.

Our auric field is like a sponge and can easily absorb the energies of those we interact with closely. Soaking up feelings and receiving others' thoughts can be an uplifting experience if we are around high-energy or positive souls,

Ultimate Self-Care

but it can also be disconcerting. This absorption can also occur to such an extent that it becomes more challenging to differentiate between our own feelings and thoughts and those belonging to someone else. This is particularly true of caregivers of family members and healers or clinicians who work with people who are ill, dying, highly anxious, or in states of anger, grief, or depression. As we develop our skills in discernment in what we are feeling and why we have those feelings, we will become more proficient in clearing our energies and knowing what feelings are actually our own.

When you suddenly feel down, sad, angry, out of sorts, or just off in some way with no immediate reason, ask yourself if these thoughts or feelings are your own or someone else's. Then wait for an inner answer to come.

If you're still not clear, you can say, "If these thoughts or feelings of [anger, despair, sadness, etc.] are not mine, then I send them out to the universe to be dissolved immediately." Then see if your mood or thoughts shift.

No matter where we are—at work, at home, in a restaurant, in a movie theatre, in a lecture hall, or on a bus or subway—we can absorb energy states of others and hold them in our own energy field. We can become easily drained, physically and emotionally, and not recognize why. If we become bogged down by the cumulative energies of others, we cannot clearly feel what our own feelings really are; it also becomes more difficult to hear our own intuitive voice, so it is important to check in and clear our energy field. The visual exercise below is a blend of various grounding and clearing exercises I have used over the years.

The Tree Root/Rose Clearing Visualization

1) Begin by sitting comfortably in a chair with both feet touching the ground. Focus on your breath. Three times, inhale a deep, slow breath (count to 8) in through your nose and out through your mouth (count to 8).

2) Mentally scan your body beginning from the bottom of your head, through your legs, to your back, front torso, arms, neck, and head. Take note of any areas of discomfort, tension, or stress. (Areas that feel to be in discomfort signal that there are likely blocked energies present that may need healing or releasing through massage, physiotherapy, acupuncture, acupressure, Reiki, or other healing methods.)

3) **Roots:** Imagine your feet have roots extending into the center of the earth. Anchor your feet's roots around the strong core of the earth and visualize the planet's life-affirming energy coming back up through your feet, then up to your legs, through to your tailbone, where you will mentally attach it.

4) **Long-Stemmed Rose**: Imagine a beautiful white long-stemmed rose above your head. Bring down pure white light from above your head, through the rose, and have it wash over and through your entire body. As a visual, this would be like standing in a shower of beautiful white energy flowing around and through every cell of your body.

5) **Golden Rose:** Imagine you have a golden-colored rose that acts like a powerful vacuum cleaner. Visualize that golden rose encircling all around your

auric field and completely sucking up any lingering energetic blobs of debris that have not been cleared away from the earlier white light. When you feel finished, visualize tossing the golden rose out into space, and see it disintegrate completely into the purity of the universe.

Clearing by Smudging

Smudging with the smoke of burning herbs, grasses, sticks of white sage, cedar, lavender, osha root, mugwort, or sweet grass is a beneficial way of cleansing away negative energies around you. Smudging comes from the First Nations or Native American healing and shamanic traditions and recognizes our connection to the sacredness of plant energies.[6]

Each plant or herb has its own unique qualities and offers up its intelligent, purifying, healing, and energizing benefits. Be aware of your intention when involved in smudging, as you connect with and honor the plant's sacred healing qualities. In essence, individually, the practice of smudging around the body for cleansing holds that when burning certain herbs, the smoke will attach itself to the negative energies. As the smoke clears, so does the negative energy that was present in the auric field.

---

[6] More information on techniques and smudging in various venues: "Indigenous Performing Arts Alliance, Smudging Document"(www.cda-acd./docs/advocacy/smudging-Document-June-2015.pdf); "Smudging Ceremony, Native American Customs & Traditions"(https://powwow-power.com/smudging/)

The result is a feeling of being refreshed and energized. This is a good practice to have before an important event or after a depleting or emotionally draining experience.

To Smudge Yourself

- Be clear about your intention to clear your mind and body of any negativity.
- Light a smudging stick (it is preferable to use a candle to light rather than a match or lighter).
- To cleanse yourself, blow out the stick and allow the stick to smolder.
- Fan the smoke with your hands or by using a feather, and go from head to foot, allowing the negative energy to flow out. Encourage it to wash over your body from atop your head, around your body, down to your feet, or vice versa.
- During this process, you can remain quiet in thought, speak your intentions, or voice a simple prayer.

The Quick Overall Body Clearing Technique

If you have been on public transportation or have been in the company of other people and want to clear your auric energy field, and your time and space limited, you can do the following in a minute or less:

Simply take both of your hands and run them just over your head, or even through your hair like a comb. Toss or

Ultimate Self-Care

flick the energy away from yourself (but not onto someone else).

Then take your hands and go down your arms, torso, and legs. Take your right hand and run it down your left arm and over your hand, and flick the excess energy off from your left hand out to the universe. Do the exact same thing with your left hand, running it down your right arm and hand and flicking it out to the universe. Imagine your hand is a dust buster, vacuum, or golden rose, and use it all around you to completely vacuum up any residual debris. Breathe deeply and put an egg-shaped oval of white light around you. Drink a glass of purified, filtered, or alkalized water.

Mind Clearing Command

There are times when our minds become preoccupied with anxious, fearful, angry, or critical thoughts. These thoughts can be about a person we have issues with or a situation we have not resolved. Sometimes, these thoughts can reflect deeper hurts, and we need more help to get them sorted out to obtain a sense of peace.

It can be very beneficial to have a method to help clear our minds, even for a short period of time. I first read about mind clearing in John Randolph Price's *The Superbeings* (1981). Understanding that our words have great power, many have used a firm statement or "command" with clear results. I have used variations of Price's statement below for many years and found it effective. Once you say it (out loud is best, but not required), wait a minute or so, and you can experience a shift to a clearer state of mind.

This statement is just an example; change the words to suit yourself. The important thing is that you know your own word is stated for your own best interests, backed up by the sincerity of your feelings, and harms no one. It therefore acts as a powerful clearing command. The "Law of Spirit," as Price states in the extrapolated version below, refers to the creative power of universal energy that surrounds us and is within us.

"I call on the Law of Spirit to clear out any thoughts in my conscious mind that resemble fear, rejection, prejudice, inadequacy, impatience, and criticism of myself or others. I don't need them, and I command them gone."

Chakra Clearing Using Musical Tones and Crystals

Music is a powerful universal language, and there is ample proof that healing tones bring about a sense of balance and rejuvenation. Specific sounds, tones, and frequencies go hand in hand with chakra clearing, balancing, and healing. We actually know this instinctively when we are drawn to the soothing tone of someone's caring voice or the calming effect of music set in tonal frequencies that bring us a sense of calm and peace.

Many health care settings, including postoperative acute care, utilize soothing vibrational music to heal, lower blood pressure, and boost immunity. We could certainly expand on using soothing tones in more of our health care settings.

Crystal singing bowls have also been used for centuries to effectively cleanse and balance chakras. I have a crystal bowl and use it when I want to feel energized and clear my mind. The sound is highly resonating, as I can feel it go

Ultimate Self-Care

through my entire body in a matter of seconds. The sound feels wonderful, and the results are immediate. Many Reiki and other energy healers use crystal bowls in their daily work.

Crystals, along with gemstones and other stones, are also alive with the energy of the universe flowing through them; their natural healing and restorative properties have been used for centuries to help clear and rebalance chakra energy centers. During their work, energy healers will often place specific crystals and stones on the chakra centers and around the body to amplify the effectiveness of the healing.

Crystals in particular, aside from being powerful in their healing capacities, are also used in countless technologies from watches to medical devices to electronics. There is a consciousness that we find when getting to know crystals, meaning that when we understand the crystal kingdom being ancient and alive with earth's evolving energy, we begin to develop a deeper relationship with their powerful energetic essence, as we would do with the other natural inhabitants of our planet.

Additional websites for healing and clearing tones can be found on Youtube. [7]

For myself, I have a natural resonance for crystals; I could never really explain why that was, except they're

---

[7] Steven Halpern, *Balancing and Healing: Meditation Music with Crystal Bowls*; *Chakra Balancing and Healing Chakra Suite: Halpern Inner Peace Music,* https://www.stevenhalpern.com; "Chakra Healing Sounds": https://balance.chakrahealing sounds.com/the-7 chakras

beautiful and seemed to have a somewhat mysterious power. Not until I began to study rocks and other gems did I understand how they were formed from volcanic magma in a specific, recognizable geometric or lattice pattern.[7] When I travelled to Egypt in 2005 with a spiritual group, I had the rare opportunity to sit in a healing circle in the King's Chamber within the Great Pyramid. I took quite a few large quartz crystals with me during that sitting, and to this day, I can feel a vibration; they are still infused with powerful energy from my time there. I offered one to a friend of mine, who could also feel this crystal vibrate in her hand.

Other books you may find helpful for understanding the precious properties and sacred uses of rocks, crystals, and minerals and their proper care are also available. [8]

Etheric Cords

Cords are really energetic, emotional attachments that we make with others or others make with us, often unconsciously. They naturally develop between us and consequentially provide speedier communication. If you are a developed clairvoyant, cords may appear to you as thin dark lines coming out of a person's body. I was able to "see", or have an inner sight of, subtle cords that were attached to one of my instructors extending outward, when I was taking a spiritual course. At that time, I was involved in various mediations and in experiencing my natural clairvoyance.

---

[8] Doreen Virtue and Judith Lukomski, *Crystal Therapy: How to Heal and Empower Your Life with Crystal Energy* (2005); Judy Hall, *The Crystal Bible* (2003); Doreen Virtue, *Chakra Clearing: Awakening Your Spiritual Power to Know and Heal* (1998).

It was not difficult to learn to see these subtle cords. I was simply required to be focused and in a meditative, relaxed state.

Energy cords between people can be connected to their specific chakra centers, depending on the nature of the relationship. For example, some cords between romantic or intimate partners are seen being attached to some of the chakras, or specifically to the heart chakra and to the second (sexual) chakra. Those attachments can be negative or positive, depending on the quality of the relationship.

Positive energy cords are natural and can be felt between those in loving relationships, such as with spouses, parents, children, close friends, and of course, animals we love. These cords run energy between people that feels uplifting and empowering.

Negative cords can also be experienced when we find ourselves in relationships with people who are connected to us through fear, depression, and anxiety. We may find these energy cords between those people addicted to substances or codependent people and their spouses or family members. This energetic attachment can be draining and leave you feeling fatigued. You can anticipate a significant energy drain as well, when a partner or family member is being abusive, manipulative, or controlling.

In the people-helping areas of work, energy cords can also attach to you from people who have been injured or traumatized, and are in states of grief. These energy attachments are not considered negative, as they form naturally, particularly in social services or health care settings where there is heavier reliance on those giving care to vulnerable people in recovery.

However, there are times when people being assisted by a practitioner or caregiver can develop a natural overattachment if their health is so compromised or they are too isolated. This client dependency can also begin to pull on the empathic heart and soul of the practitioner, as has been my experience, having been in counseling roles many times. It is necessary to know the various ways to clear yourself and stay uplifted, not only to provide your best support to others, but to ensure you have enough energy for your own personal life.

If you experience a drain on your energy that requires a small break or even a greater separation from someone or a situation, you may find the next section on cord cutting useful. You don't need to feel you are being negative in doing this; you only need to be aware that you are doing something out of self-regard, in respecting that you are responsible for taking good care of your own energy, by mindfully detaching from someone else's energy attachment.

Cord Cutting

Cord cutting is one of the ways we can detach with love and respectfully assist in clearing and supporting ourselves. People who work extensively with others, not just professionals but *anyone* who is caring for others in any capacity, can use cord cutting daily as a matter of routine to keep their energy clear.

Importantly, cord cutting does not destroy a relationship that still has growth involved, but it does serve to energetically eradicate unhealthy aspects of energy between people while maintaining the true loving connection. The love that truly

Ultimate Self-Care

exists between people is never destroyed because it is the energy that exists throughout all time.

However, if it's best to be disconnected from that person, the intelligent spiritual energy you call upon will assist in creating more of a severance, according to your best interests. Be aware that when you cut cords, you may also find those people you are detaching from can psychically pick up the detachment without conscious understanding. They may feel a sudden need to reconnect. To keep the disconnection intact, be prepared to set any needed boundaries should they contact you. The section on boundaries that follows in this chapter can be helpful in this process.

Cord Cutting Exercise

Ground and center yourself in whatever method works best for you. One way is to sit in a comfortable chair and imagine a silver cord from your spine going deep into the earth and anchoring you at the planet's core; this is a quick way to use imagery for grounding.

Take a moment to again breathe deeply, inhale and exhale slowly three times, and think of the person you want to clear or create distance from.

Think of a large pair of scissors and imagine them cutting all cords that are around you, beneath your feet and above your head.

Imagine your surrounding auric energy field as clean and unattached from this person. As you release this person, ask that this person be blessed by love, spirit, or whoever, or whatever you may wish to name. You can also imagine pink light going toward them and surrounding them; bless them in their life's journey.

You can say to yourself, "I release [name] from my life, and I am thankful for the lessons I take with me. It is done, and I am free."

Your words and your natural ability to visualize create a powerful command. Remembering this allows us to be mindful of what we say and how we say it (negative thoughts create negative energy, and vice versa).

Clearing and Raising Home or Workspace Energy

With so many systemic changes and challenges, stresses can lead to feelings of frustration, moodiness, fear, and negativity. Combine those challenges with the smaller home spaces we live in, as well as smaller pod areas in which many people find themselves working so closely together, and the result is a more pronounced buildup of negative energy. It is good to clear and raise our home or workspace energy.

Negative energy gets stuck in cluttered places because clutter creates energy blocks. It gets stuck in our home and workspaces when tragedy or sadness builds up from the serious, traumatic, and depressing situations we face. For those who work in helping professions, or parents and adult children who care for loved ones, or who have helped another through tragedy, there is a real need to debrief about their experiences. Even though it is beneficial in the moment, the energy in that emotional sharing is still discharged into the environment and can remain. All thoughts, words, and feelings are forms of energy and can be imprinted into our environment: the walls, chairs, rugs, whatever is visible or not-so-visible. It all remains there until we consciously clear it away.

Strategies to clear and raise the vibrational levels in our home or work environments involve our human energetic selves, in that our own frequencies in the end ultimately give rise to improved home or workspace feelings. We are energy beings, and we use forms of energy. Everything is connected in some way. The following suggestions can affect us more personally and also positively impact the environment:

Decluttering

First, look to your own home or workspace and see if there is anything you can clear, reorganize, or declutter. At work, it is not surprising to see one colleague clearing her/his space followed by others. Setting the example can be psychologically encouraging because we instinctively know we feel better and work better in an organized space, even if it only lasts for a few days, and we have to go at it again. Decluttering should be done on a routine basis as a habit to make the positive energy setting in your home or work feel best for you.

Smudging the Environment

In a broader measure, it is useful to explore the use of smudging in your home or workspace. We know this is an effective way of clearing our body's auric field, and it can assist in clearing an environment. It's a good idea is to smudge yourself individually before doing an environmental smudge.

- Be clear about your intention to cleanse your space of negativity and follow the same process of lighting your herb.
- Pay attention to allowing smoke into corners, behind doors, in closet spaces, around windows, and even around electronics. You may also want to look into a smudging spray to better serve your purposes, rather than using smoke.
- As above, during your individual smudge, you can remain quiet in thought, speak your intentions, or voice a simple prayer.
- You can do this process of clearing your space as an individual, or as a group, or splitting a group off into several areas.

Power in the Voice

As we're aware of specific vibrational tones to calm, heal, clear, and energize, we can also consider many benefits in using our voices, singularly or collectively, to raise our personal vibration and energy, and extend that positivity to our home and workspaces by singing or chanting. The combination of sound, breath, and rhythm, when practiced consistently, changes our neurological systems and shifts and rebalances our mind-body connections toward increased soothing, calmness, and a sense of well-being.

The elation that arises from singing is from a release of endorphins or oxytocin, both associated with pleasure.

In short, singing can be transformative. It is no surprise that singing is reported on the rise, as it can literally and figuratively contribute to an overall harmonizing of people and environments. Group singing is no longer the domain of church choirs. There are many types of singing groups springing up throughout areas of work and community living.

"Singing Improves Health and Work Environment" (*Science Nordic*, Nov. 12, 2012) reported that employees in two hospitals in Norway decided on a project called the Sound of Well-Being, to see the impact of singing on its employees. There were two groups: employees who participated and those who did not. The overall finding was that those employees who participated in the singing groups reported a higher commitment to their workplace than their non-singing colleagues, with an additional self-assessed improvement in their health over those who didn't participate. The speed of the bonding pointed to a faster cohesion between unfamiliar individuals, resulting in what researchers Pearce, Launay, and Dunbar (2015) called the "ice-breaker effect of singing."

CBC News (2015) (https://www.cbc.ca/news/health/choir-sing-bond-1.3367438) reported that "choirs offer fast ice-breaker effect to foster social bonds," citing a music-as-medicine study that revealed classmates over a seven-month period at the University of Oxford's adult education courses bonded quickest through singing as compared to creative writing or crafts.

These positive vibrations extending out into our surrounding physical environment have other beneficial impacts. Prolific research being done by Dr. Monica Gagliano from the University of Western Australia sees plants as living, dynamic sentient beings. She has extensively studied the intelligent relationship among plants, animals, and humans using sound, and she continuously hums and plays music to her plants. (https://www.monicagagliano.com).

Drumming

As most people know, nearly every culture in the world has practiced some form of drumming. Shamans and healers worldwide recognize drumming's holistic healing benefits. Drumming is also closely associated with First Nations peoples; some have referred to drumming as being the heartbeat of Mother Earth.

Drumming has been significantly used for healing, during meditation, and in spiritual, social, political, and civic ceremonies. You'll notice that the beat of the drum provides the backbone of a song's rhythm; the even metric beat grounds the music and allows the creative instruments to flow.

Drumming as a stand-alone experience also has the same benefits that singing has but is more noteworthy for lowering blood pressure and stress through the act of hitting and hearing the beat. It can even become quickly meditative through repetition.

Drum circles are inclusive events for all age groups that can involve just drumming or can also incorporate singing, body percussion (striking the body to produce sounds), and guided imagery. Levitin and Chandra (2013, 179) acknowledged that overall, music positively affects brain chemistry and mental health function by aiding in stress reduction, boosting immunity, managing mood, and assisting in social bonding. Most specifically, drumming circles for seniors actually reversed some age-related deterioration.

In Vancouver, BC, facilitator Lyle Povah (2011), who researched a drum circle program for eating disorders at Saint Paul's Hospital, said that "in the health care environment, drum circles promote self-expression and self-empowerment. Following drum circles, patients report feeling more energized, relaxed and joyful."

In a well-known study by Dr. Barry Bittman (2001, 38–47), the American neurologist introduced drumming in a Pennsylvania senior nursing home over six weeks to research the benefits of drumming. He saw a 50 percent increase in staff mood and a decrease in depression and fatigue among residents. He said, "Group drumming tunes our biology, orchestrates our immunity, and enables healing to begin."

There has been a resurgence of drumming circles for all ages and across all societal areas, including the corporate world. During the summer months on some local beaches in British Columbia, for example, you will hear the rhythmic, joyful, and enticing sounds of djembe and conga drums in the evening, bringing all ages together.

Using Color to Influence Energy

I consciously pick colors for my daily self-care to boost my energy, convey an impression, or simply help me feel emotionally comfortable. Color is important to us in where we live, what we wear, and how we feel. Colors also connect

Barbara Halcrow, MSW

us. For example, I tend toward bolder, brighter, non-pastel colors. When I am giving a presentation, I resonate to wearing darker blue colors, especially royal blue, because I have always felt blue was a spiritual color for me and connects with how I am feeling and helps me to express myself. Red is useful for an immediate energy hit and is a good color; if I'm in an emotionally challenging situation, I'll wear a calmer mauve or purple color, instead. Bright yellow or orange hues go well in adding to a quiet energy and inspiration, and I often wear black in the evening to add an air of sophistication.

An interesting phenomenon I've witnessed in workplaces is after several months of getting to know people, several of us will turn up wearing the same color on the same day. Sometimes these colors reflect the colors of the upper chakras in their emotional and spiritual colors of green, blue, violet, or purple hues, making a simple demonstration of the closer emotional and spiritual links between us.

Color was widely recognized for centuries by the ancients and Indigenous peoples across continents for its importance in spiritual meaning, symbolism, and ceremony. The use of colors encompasses many areas of our lives, involving sacred aspects in diverse religions, spiritual beliefs, and cultural and ceremonial practices and healings (Wills 1993).

The colors we wear, what we see in nature, and what we surround ourselves with in our homes and working environments all act to influence us in mind, body, and spirit, as well as our behavior. Animals and plants are also affected by color, and each color also has its own vibration and measurable wavelength (Chambers 2016).

Ultimate Self-Care

When we begin with the natural light from the sun at dawn and continue through to the darkness of night after sunset, we are experiencing the powerful effects of the rainbow of colors contained in this electromagnetic spectrum of light from the sun. This light is akin to the same electromagnetic waves as radio and television signals, and light is the natural part of the spectrum we can actually see. This natural light is made up of the primary colors of red, orange, yellow, green, blue, and violet.

We can see the primary colors when we allow light to flow through a prism and those colors fall into the rainbow pattern, or when we see a natural rainbow in the sky as light is dispersed and reflected through the droplets of water.

To consciously use color as an energy tool for self-care, we can first pay attention to what colors we are drawn to, as well as when we are drawn to them and how we feel. Each color has its own energy vibration that has an impact on us. Some colors will energize and invigorate us, soothe and calm us, or put us on alert. All colors have a dual psychological impression of negative and positive, depending on what mood and situation we are in, and what message about ourselves we want to convey.

Traditionally, cross-culturally, spiritually, there can also be differences attributed to each color. For example, in Western societies, black can symbolize formality and sophistication or dark and evil energy. In Egyptian culture, black can be associated with rebirth and transformation, and in Africa, the color can represent maturation, particularly for males (Wills 1993, Wang 2015).

Some colors included below will have similarities corresponding to chakra and auric colors. The list below reflects the main colors we tend to think of the most in Western society.

Black: Black represents all colors absorbed into one; therefore, there is an absence of light. Black can bring in a sense of authority, protection, glamour, or sophistication. Conversely, it can also represent heaviness, coldness, a threat, or even oppression. If you are already feeling down, black may not be your best choice. If you choose to lighten it up, some of the more energetic colors below can help.

Brown: Brown is a natural, earthy color that represents reliability, groundedness, and warmth. Brown can also initially convey an impression of humility or sometimes of being too serious. This color can be helpful to soften, stabilize, and ground your energy.

Gray: Gray can be experienced as a neutral color. It's not always best in exuding confidence, unless you accent it with a brighter color, as it doesn't express as much energy or vitality. Silver is actually gray with a metallic or polished sheen. This color can help you to appear businesslike, but it may lack a sense of warmth you might want to convey.

Red: Red is a strong color, as it is most often connected to our physical senses, giving arousal to feelings of strength, passion, and vitality. It can also awaken us to possible alarm, such as in the case of stoplights, police lights, or ambulance lights. Wear red to increase your energy; you will undoubtedly stand out. Red can also be interpreted as a more assertive color. Some people can be intimidated if you wear red, while others will be drawn to your vitality and self-confidence.

Pink: Pink is actually a tint derivative of red, but it has a far more soothing effect on us, especially the pastel pinks, which are often seen as the more feminine, romantic, softer color against the more culturally active or masculinized color of red. Fortunately, our traditional, restrictive concepts of gender have become more expansive, and colors are also being used in a more expressive way, particularly by North American men.

Orange: Orange plays more into our sense of fun, comfort, warmth, and sensuality. It can help awaken our creativity. Orange is red and yellow combined. Some color specialists suggest that given the expansive nature of orange, it's good to combine it with a cooler color, such as blue, for balance.

Yellow: Yellow is seen as the strongest stimulating psychological color, as its wavelength is long. One can experience optimism, emotional and intellectual strength, and extroversion when wearing or seeing this color. As with orange, a combined cooler color like blue or black is good for strength in balance. Gold is metallic yellow, or a yellow hue can also be referred to as golden.

Green: Green is a color whose impression is one of harmony, balance, love, healing, and peace. It is located in the center of the color spectrum and makes us feel closer to nature and all of her abundance. It can be calming and quietly energizing, simultaneously, and it is often used in healing or medical centers to help people relax. Darker greens can impress as being wealthy. As an opposite impression, green can be seen as unmoving or even stagnate, or when associated with food, rancid.

Blue: Blue is perceived to be an intellectual color and gives rise to positive and efficient communication, calm, and coolness. Many people, including myself, will wear blue near our throat chakra when wanting to ensure clear communications. Blue is often worn for job interviews, as it symbolizes loyalty. Contrasting impressions of blue can leave one feeling too cool, unemotional, unfeeling, or aloof.

Purple or Violet: These synonymous colors are most often connected to our sense of spirituality, spiritual awareness, truth, and inner vision. This color, depending on the hue, can both liven up your energy as well as create an impression of introversion and deeper thought.

White: White is the complete opposite of black and is a total reflection of all colors. It is often not so easy to look at white and is characterized as pure, hygienic, simple, sophisticated, standoffish, and elite.

The information discussed above has been extrapolated from several websites and texts that give detailed information on the influence of colors.[9]

As we saw throughout this chapter, there are many ways we can ground, clear, and raise our energies; we sometimes do these things quite instinctively. Paying attention to all our senses and nourishing ourselves as best as possible can be an exploration that becomes deeply meaningful.

---

[9] Angela Wright, *Psychological Colours of Properties, Colour Affects* (2008–2016), http://www.colour-affects.co.uk/psychological-properties-of-colours; David Johnson, *Colour Psychology: Do Different Colours Affect Your Mood?* (2000–2016), https://www.infoplease.com/color-psychology; Susana Martinex-Conde, Stephen L. Machknik, "How the Colour Red Influences Our Behaviour," *Scientific America, Behaviour and Society* (January 11, 2014), https://www.scientificamerican.com/article/ho-the-color-red-influences-our-behviour/; Pauline Wills, "Colour Therapy" in *Health Essentials: The Use of Colour for Health and Healing.* Great Britain: Element Books, 1993.

Supporting ourselves with kindness, care, and consideration is a demonstration of self-love.

The next chapter will look at various ways we can effectively and gently protect all our energy systems, beginning with our body's outer auric field.

CHAPTER 4

PROTECTING YOUR ENERGY

Your Surrounding Energy Field

Protecting your energy field is about setting a boundary. As you set emotional and physical boundaries, it's a good idea to also set a boundary around your entire auric field; I will expand on that below. Using your mental and visual capabilities is an important part of protecting yourself in the unseen realm. Later in this chapter, we will also look at boundaries more closely connected to the emotional and physical body.

Over the years, I have come to recognize that I am a very strong empath; people who are empathic experience their feelings on a deep level, and they are also very tuned into the feelings and emotional states of others around them, including animals. We are very sponge-like. Constantly absorbing other people's feelings—particularly those feelings of fear, anger, sadness, or depression—has an overall deleterious impact, in that these feelings will begin to feel like they are our very own. They can also amplify our own inner sadness, grief, and anger. Though we cannot avoid feeling what others feel—and we should not be afraid of doing that, for that is the beauty of our sensitivity as humans—we can still offer ourselves some protection as to the impact of this level of absorption. We can use visualization as a tool to assist us.

Admittedly, this is an area of vulnerability for me, as I do pick up and absorb people's energy, and I often forget to use protective energy visuals. I tend to mostly use clearing techniques for my energy, when I feel I need to. However, I would be remiss in discussing this area with you. Some of my spiritual colleagues do not believe in the concept of protecting your energy, but some do. I give this information to you, as the reader, to use as you feel it suits you.

You can clear your auric field first by following the clearing exercises provided in chapter 3, or use some other exercise you prefer. You can also try the visualization below using white and violet light, which also act as a clearing energy.

Exercise: The Egg and the Color of Violet

1. **Focus on your breath** and inhale a deep slow breath (count from 1 to 4) in through your nose and then out through your mouth (count from 1 to 4). Do this breathing three times.
2. **Imagine pure white light** descending from above your crown center over your body and through your body, down into the ground. Imagine it clearing out your auric field of unwanted negative thoughts or feelings, as well as from your inner chakras and any other cells of the body. Imagine it is now gently enwrapping you and covering your entire auric energy field like a giant egg, strong and protective in its very nature and shape. The egg shape is a loving symbol of earth and of life.

Ultimate Self-Care

3. **When you have finished,** and if you want to add an extra layer of protection, think about the color violet. Violet can be used as a protective color; it's an alchemic color of transmutation. I have used this color myself and feel that of the various colors I've used over the years, this has felt the most powerful for me. I am also very tuned in to this color and feel it really does align well with my higher spiritual nature. Violet has origins that go back centuries, with powerful connections to the ascended master, Saint Germain.

4. **Imagine this violet color** now becomes a violet flame, gently flowing down through all your chakras and cells as well as over your entire auric field, covering the protective egg shape you created. The violet flame is another very powerful transmuter of negative energies. Besides shielding yourself, you can use it to shield animals, other people, items, and even places. You can command that this violet flame cleanse all negativity from your mind, body, and spirit and protect your energy system.

I have used the formal invocations for the violet flame in my past meditative/spiritual practices. I will respectfully leave it for the reader, if interested, to acquire more understanding of this powerful realm and expansive use of the violet flame for protecting, transmuting, and healing energies; there are other resources cited below. [10]

---

[10] E. C. Prophet, *The Violet Flame to Heal Body, Mind and Soul* (Summit Publications, Inc., 1997); *The Violet Flame*; *The Secret of the Violet Flame,* 2016, http://violetflame.com/violet-flame-secret/

Barbara Halcrow, MSW

Your Intention

I believe it bears repeating that the power of any of these protective measures lies in your clear and mindful intention to create them. We can all develop our own protective energy shields, because the power of our mental images, our words, and our beliefs are so strong as to be completely integral to our outer experiences being formed or cocreated. In other words, what lies inside may eventually manifest outside.

Invocations

There are other ways to give us protection. Some people invoke the angelic realm or other spiritual figures or guides known to them. Again, it's your own preference in what works for you. There are many documented stories about this powerful spiritual level of beings that defy normal human explanation.

There are now countless worldwide first-person reports of sudden encounters with the physical appearance of strangers who appear out of nowhere and offer life-saving assistance, from unseen hands pulling people from disastrous situations to sudden warnings that prevent injuries or death.

One reference is *Proof of Angels* by Ptolemy Tompkins and Tyler Beddoes (2016), and another is John Geiger's book, *The Angel Effect* (2013). These authors have collected first-hand accounts from hundreds of offerings that tell of amazing and miraculous interventions. I experienced my own divine interventions that I strongly believe were the result of this higher realm stepping in, with virtually no time to spare, to intervene and save my life.

Ultimate Self-Care

One example of divine intervention was when I was travelling with a friend down a canyon highway and was making a sharp turn on the road, only to find a bus suddenly bearing down on us. It appeared in that split-second to have crossed into our lane; the bus was so close, it filled up our entire front window. Suddenly, there was a bright flash that blocked my sight, like someone took a flash camera and you couldn't see anything for a second or two. The next instant, we were still driving on the highway, but the bus now appeared far back in my rearview mirror. I felt stunned, and neither of us could speak for a several seconds to acknowledge that something supernatural had just occurred. I knew that our lives had been spared, and there was no explanation for it, except that an intervening, loving presence had stepped in to save us.

Authors such as Dianna Cooper, Lorna Byrne, and Dr. William Bloom have spent years giving detailed instruction and guidance as to how this powerful spiritual domain works, including how each person's personal guardian angel can assist in any area of our daily lives.

However, as with any situation, looking within ourselves first—to our instinctive, gut sense as well as our basic common sense—can bring us important and immediate impressions, answers, and insights, which allow us greater degrees of safety and help us avoid unwanted consequences.

If, though, you want to invoke the angelic realm for protection, you can make this request of your guardian angels in any situation. Of the archangels, Michael is recognized as the most powerful in offering protection: emotionally, spiritually, and physically. This archangel's attributes are courage, strength, truth, and integrity. Simply ask mentally or verbally for Archangel Michael's assistance. Ultimately, it is up to you and what you choose to believe in, because our personal beliefs hold potent power behind any request.

Generally speaking, the power of our own spoken word cannot be underestimated, as it acts as a powerful command to the universal, intelligent energy we all have access to, to cocreate with us exactly what we are asking for (discussed in more detail in chapter 5).

The Importance of Our Personal Boundaries

> *The most important distinction anyone can ever make in their life is between who they are as an individual and their connection with others.*
>
> —Anné Linden

There are many different kinds of boundaries in our society. With regard to knowledge of our personal boundaries, few children are taught the importance of knowing and asserting those core limits. We come from varying degrees of dysfunctional family backgrounds and often learn about our boundaries and our personal protective rights after they have been crossed.

Yet boundaries are one of the most important things that define our identities and help keep us safe. Boundaries tell others what we value, what we believe in, how we choose to govern our lives, and how we want others to treat us. Essentially, there are four main boundary areas: physical boundaries, emotional boundaries, mental boundaries, and spiritual boundaries.

Physical Boundaries

Our physical boundaries, in terms of the degree of space in which we like to feel safe and comfortable, can be part of our cultural heritage as well as the nature of our friendships and intimate relationships. Other more obvious physical boundaries involve our personal spaces at home or at work, as well as our range of personal belongings.

Barbara Halcrow, MSW

An example of an important physical boundary revolves around touch. This is sometimes a confusing area for those who have been violated as children, as example, and have never healed from that violation. Other people assume they are entitled to touch others as they wish, without permission. Unwanted touching can reflect racism, sexism, and abuse of one's power and control. If you are not sure if someone has crossed this boundary with you, check in with yourself to see how you feel. If you recoil or experience a sense of being uncomfortable, then trust your feelings that your boundary was crossed.

Emotional Boundaries

Having a clear sense of how we feel about what is important to us, while at the same time being able to respectfully appreciate where someone else is at, even if we don't always agree, strikes a good balance for healthy emotional boundaries. For example, I may hold fast that I do not feel emotionally safe with a certain individual someone else may be perfectly comfortable spending time with, and I will need to accept the other's feelings, without voicing criticism, judging, or resorting to gossip. Another example is that I may not enjoy music that others love to hear; it might be too loud, boring, or irritating to me. That's fine, and I may need to choose to say something about my preference or adjust spending my time with them should it be a constant irritation. Being able to disagree and assert our feelings and not cave into being manipulated (or manipulating others) is also part of having healthy emotional boundaries.

If we feel taken for granted and there is a pattern evolving, that may be seen as having our emotional boundaries crossed. This is when our expressed needs and wants are ignored, or we don't feel listened to or accepted for who we are. Respecting our own needs and wishes as being as valuable as those of others, and being able to state our own needs and wants clearly, is necessary for healthy, interdependent relationships.

Verbal name-calling, insults, or disrespectful language directed at you or anyone else is also a clear example of abuse of our emotional boundaries. With healthy emotional boundaries, we can independently meet more of our own emotional needs without relying on someone else.

This move toward a greater sense of self as being whole and complete as we are helps strengthen us and keeps our emotional attachments from becoming overly dependent, as in addictive or codependent relationships. Since the world we live in promotes addictions and overattachments every which way possible, gaining a greater independent, whole, and complete self is a lengthy, evolving process.

Mental Boundaries

Mental boundaries are different from our emotional boundaries. Mental boundaries are about how we think and reason and come to our own conclusions about how we live, what we value, and just about anything we choose to believe. When people try to insert their opinions or thoughts into our mind frame, attempting to manipulate us, control us, or make us feel guilty or emotionally responsible for their behavior, then we are being signaled that our mental boundaries are being crossed. Our minds are likely being manipulated. We can choose to assert our thoughts and opinions in respectful ways without intruding on others.

Spiritual Boundaries

Spiritual boundaries can be connected to our mental and emotional boundaries. Spiritual boundaries can also be perceived in different ways by many people, depending sociocultural factors. For example, we all have personal views of the Creator, God, Goddess, Allah, Buddha, our Higher Self, or some guiding energy in our spiritual lives. It is not for anyone else to determine or pressure us to acknowledge anything other than what feels right for us. If we do not believe in anything as being spiritually relevant to us, that is also valid and acceptable. Spiritual boundary development can also involve those we agree to associate with who share similar thoughts, beliefs, feelings, and views on life, as well as their personal conduct. It's an area of our overall discernment that requires a thoughtful approach.

Spiritual boundaries can also involve being mindful of not giving others unsolicited clairvoyant or any other form of intuitive spiritual assessment or readings without having the subject's or a third party's permission. This area can feel complicated, but if there is ever a doubt as a spiritual advisor or reader, the advisor can help the client rephrase a potentially invasive question such as, "Is my partner having an affair?" to "What do I need to know about this situation, and in what ways can I best manage myself?" In that way, there is a spiritual and ethical boundary put in place. (Generally, going within ourselves to seek answers is a good practice overall, and learning to use tarot, oracle cards, rune stones, I Ching, or other forms of divination can be useful.)

Good Boundaries Exude Strength

When you know what your boundaries are, people become instinctively aware of that fact because you will exude an unspoken strength. This strength acts as a deterrent to others who tend to practice control and manipulation. Your energy is not attractive to them. This strength also lets people know you are respectful of their boundaries as well.

Good boundaries help you to say no or yes in various circumstances that require you to regulate all manner of people, situations, and demands that enter your life. Unregulated demands and stresses can become overwhelming. We see evidence of this in people who are overextended, leading to staff burnout in social service and health care arenas. This energy exhaustion and burnout can occur from the front line, to middle management, and up to the director's level.

The ability to consciously regulate the stimuli in your personal as well as your daily work life will also allow you to feel more confident and express yourself in a more authentic way. Your realness will pull in more of the respect you deserve. You will also attract better personal and work-life circumstances because respecting yourself draws respect from others. We are constantly teaching people how to treat us.

If you've not practiced being definitive before, defining and standing up for your boundaries in personal relationships will bring challenges from family, friends, or even ex-partners. It can surprise people who may have enjoyed receiving your attention in a manner that no longer serves you. In short, they probably won't be too happy about your stand for clarity and limit setting, and you may ultimately receive comments to suggest your attitude needs a serious adjustment. Just stand firm in your decision to support your true worth and uphold what you most treasure: yourself.

Know Yourself

The better we know ourselves in as many areas as possible, the easier it is to set our boundaries and limits. That doesn't mean that knowing ourselves will suddenly create the balance we need for home and work challenges and our own necessary self-care, but it will definitely help.

Over the course of a hectic or chaotic day, you sometimes lose clarity about yourself, and in those moments, you need to take time to go inward, take a few breaths, and reflect on how you really feel to re-establish some clarity around your time and space. In those moments, just remember to sit quietly and breathe in and out. This will immediately begin to quiet your mind for clearer inner listening. You can use any of the grounding, clearing, and protection measures you've read about.

The clarity that comes from practice in focusing on your feelings, wishes, and nourishment needs is important to setting good boundaries. It is also good to have a sense of your own pace regarding how fast or slow you like to do things. If someone makes a request of your time, and you're not sure about that request, establish for yourself how much time you have left in a day (automatically include a few moments for yourself), and then pace more slowly in terms of what kind of time is actually realistic for you to give, and in what manner and context.

Setting Boundaries

Setting boundaries means clarifying and making mindful, informed decisions about how to prioritize your time around work, family members, friends, and other activities, as well as making it a priority to spend as much nourishing self-care time as possible with yourself. Remember to do the following:

- Clearly know and speak your limits to those around you
- Support your boundaries or limit setting with healthy decisions that nourish your well-being
- Try to maintain consistency in your responses
- Remember that your self-respecting actions teach others how to treat you

Saying No and Feeling Guilty

If you set a boundary and feel guilty, that's not a bad sign. It generally means you are resetting the expectations of yourself and others that may have kept you in place and even entrapped you. It's an emotional adjustment process, and it takes time and patience.

Setting personal boundaries and sticking to them while others complain that their needs are not being met can initially feel selfish or self-centered, but it's really about honoring and respecting yourself. People don't often like change, especially when they experience you as taking yourself away from meeting their needs or abandoning them. However, they'll have to get used to the new you and adjust themselves accordingly. This is where codependent or simply unhealthy, unbalanced relationships show up.

You may realize you have been an over-functioning participant, as many of us are, for periods of time. Moving away from this caregiving or rescuing role will bring you more vitality and focus to accomplish more of what matters to you.

Your life's mission and passions will also reveal themselves more clearly to you after you successfully make emotional and psychological room for them to be heard from within. Some boundaries are nonnegotiable, resulting in a strict do-not-cross boundary setting. Overall, it's important to know what boundaries are so important for you to safeguard that they are not to be tampered with at any cost.

Assertiveness Exercise

This exercise is meant to help you start the process of thinking assertively to draw in more strength from any measure of past success. Thinking about self-assertion is the first step to getting your frame of mind to back you up, followed by seeking out more help, if necessary, toward taking action to accomplish your goal.

Ultimate Self-Care

Think of a time in your life that you felt the strongest in terms of following a path you knew was clearly right for you. You can be any age, even as a child. Think of your deep commitment to following your plan through. How did you accomplish your goal? Who was there to support you? What was in place to assist you?

- Think of any measure of happiness, sense of pride, or degree of accomplishment that you experienced along the way. See if you can also recall somewhere inside yourself when you felt decisive in saying, "I *will* move forward" to whoever or whatever stood in the way of your success. Feel again your commitment to stand your ground and move yourself forward.
- Think of a present situation that is bothering you or a habit you want to be free of that is not supporting your health. Draw up your past memory and allow the strength that you had inside of you then to come forward into this present situation. Really get into the mind-set of yourself in that past time, and recall your commitment to succeed.
- Stay in that mind-set and write down any words that come to you about how you felt. Know that as soon as you put your mind in that same frame from your past, you are already on the right track to accomplishing this goal.
- Picture yourself standing strong in your commitment to assert yourself. See yourself stepping away from the current situation or negative behavior.

Assertive Bill of Rights

Develop your own list of assertiveness rights. See the list below, replicated from Gael Lindenfield,[11] a leading personal development trainer in the United Kingdom, and look at it as a psychological and emotional boost. This list can be a helpful reminder to carry with you or keep where it's easy to see.

- The right to ask for what we want, realizing that the other person has the right to say no.
- The right to have opinions, feelings, and emotions and to express them appropriately.
- The right to make statements that have no logical basis and that we don't have to justify.
- The right to make our own decisions and to cope with their consequences.
- The right to choose whether to get involved with the problems of someone else or not.
- The right to know about something or understand it.
- The right to make mistakes.
- The right to be successful.
- The right to change our mind.
- The right to privacy.
- The right to be alone and independent.
- The right to change ourselves and be more assertive.

---

[11] Gael Lindenfeld (http://www.gaellindenfield.com)

Exercise: "Would I Allow My Inner Child into This Situation?"

This question can be used by anyone to bring forward any feelings about whether a situation is safe or unsafe. It is a very useful question for those are familiar with the concept of their inner child, a term used in aspects of psychological healing work to bring us back to the wisdom or playfulness of our younger self. We can also experience our inner child when we are frightened or vulnerable. Your inner child will give you a gut sense or intuitive messages about what is safe or not safe or comfortable. Those feelings are worth listening to.

To get in touch with your inner child, picture yourself as you were when you were about eight years old. Now you, in your adult state, are the protective parent of the younger you who stands before you. You agree that you will always take care of your inner child, as best as you can, and will not force the child into unsafe or unhealthy situations. Your responsibility is to always try to make the right decision on behalf of this child. This includes always checking in to listen to the child as to how he or she is feeling, particularly in moments of stress, anxiety, fear, or uncertainty. Hug your little kid and tell her or him, "I am here for you now, and I love you."

In sum, when you choose to assert limits and boundaries to protect and nourish yourself, that reflects careful self-regard in how you expend your personal energy; this also helps others around you. Although there can be times when you are met with resistance to changes you decide to make, your self-strengthening can encourage everyone connected to you to recognize the necessity to strengthen their abilities to meet their own needs.

There are many other good resources on boundary development. [12]

---

[12] Jan Black and Greg Enns, *Better Boundaries: Owning and Treasuring Your Life* (1997); the Self Help Alliance, University of Alberta. "Building Better Boundaries" (https://cloudfront.ualberta.ca/-/media/medicine/departments/anesthesiology/documents/workbookbuilding-better-boundariesfeb2011.pdf)

CHAPTER 5

MINDFUL COMMUNICATIONS

Mind is a flexible mirror; adjust it to see a better world.

—Amit Ray

The Conscious Mind

To fully care for ourselves, we need to also care for our minds and understand what affects our mental state, positively and otherwise. Collins New English Dictionary (1999) defines *mindful* as "being aware and objective and taking into account." Being mindful of what is going on in our thoughts and feelings in various moments, without judgment or criticism, further cultivates a consciousness to accept ourselves, with compassion, in the full range of our humanness, appreciating that we are all learning and evolving on our own personal paths.

Becoming more mindful is not always easy, as there are countless daily distractions. It takes practice and vigilance over a lifetime. Becoming more consciously aware and mindful will contribute to taking far more control over our thoughts and feelings; we will be more peaceful and balanced in all our energy systems. This increased inner peace and balance will be reflected in experiencing the world in more peaceful ways.

Before we can get to the kind of Zen-like state we'd like, there can be moments where it seems we are at the mercy of our thoughts, and that's unpleasant if those thoughts are negative or fearful. Being immediately aware of the influences behind those thoughts will also help us know how we communicate our inner experiences to others and then make changes as necessary toward more peaceful interactions.

Default to the Negative

Though most people want to remain positive and hopeful, we do have a human tendency to default to the negative, where we assume the worst in people or see situations from a fearful, negative standpoint. Defaulting to the negative can also be part of a learned habit. We can fall into this tendency when we hear ourselves jumping to conclusions and, if there is something positive to consider, we ignore or invalidate it.

This tendency can also be rooted in past hurts or traumas that emerge when triggered by a comment from someone that reminds us of that negative time. Listening to our self-talk can give us a clue as to how quickly we turn to perceive situations in a pessimistic light, or if we are able to step back and think more critically to see a fuller picture.

Some researchers, like Graham (2013, 39–41), think this negativity bias of the brain toward mistrust, worry, or gloom is a hardwired evolutionary pattern, as a result of past survival issues meant to keep us alert for our survival. It can also be referred to as our "reptilian brain" (Deepak and Tanzi 2012). The reptilian brain is the part of our brain that is shared by the animals on our planet and involves

Ultimate Self-Care

instinctual triggers leading to fear and fight-or-flight reactions. The reptilian brain also creates the need to want to group together, to feel safer and stronger for maximum protection, with a focus on defending our perceived territory (Ibid., 112–17).

At present, with sociopolitical, economic, and environmental changes occurring on a global level, there is greater instability being experienced en masse, and it is triggering a resurgence of our reptilian brain.

That being said, there are a lot of sad and frightening things going on in this world that are continuously and negatively influencing our collective perceptions. Unless we are consciously aware and trained to the contrary, when our thoughts are exposed to this kind of negative information, it can make us more fearful, more vulnerable, and we pay even closer attention to the psychologically darker, weightier information that crosses our path. Fear can be contagious, but so can kindness, caring, and compassion. I believe we are more emotionally vulnerable and sensitive than we realize, and therefore, we can be emotionally influenced by what we hear and see. It is up to us know our limits around what information to allow in and how long to attend to it.

We can choose to be aware of this easy default tendency and watch incoming information with discernment. We can turn our mind's attention toward more positive, balanced, solution-focused, and uplifting thoughts, without completely denying the difficult realities occurring on this planet. We can choose to seek out positive stories about people helping people, animals, and the earth. We can choose to be aware and to open other doors to more hope, love, and kindness.

Barbara Halcrow, MSW

Media Watch

We can choose from some excellent journalistic reporting as well as thoughtful and informative programming on a global level. We have our favorite sports, comedies, reality TV, dramas, and everything else in between. Having more programming also means there is more news and likely more violence to sift through.

Negative thoughts coming in produce negative thoughts going out. Mainstream and alternative media outlets are aware of how people tend toward drama, fear, and gossip. Media also includes all manner of information streaming on the Internet. All of this communication systemically impacts us with overt and subliminal messages. Images and themes in movies, TV news, tabloid magazines, and digital games have the power to shape our perceptions and affect our feelings; they can even result in depressing physical effect on us if its content is negative.

It's truly dreadful to know about the suffering and abuse in our world, through war and other forms of death and despair. The onslaught of images and information on a daily basis creates a powerful impression that our world is a negative and unsafe place to be. Perhaps we can say with a degree of certainty that some kinds of information and images being disseminated from various outlets can become remarkably addictive, as in a type of fear porn, as the general public becomes emotionally desensitized to violence and images of death. As this desensitization continues, we are pulled away from our gentle heartedness and risk leaving behind our inner sense that tells us something isn't right about all of this.

Ultimate Self-Care

We are also seeing the advent of more fake news. Such was the case in the lead-up to the 2016 election in the United States, where much of the population in the United States, Canada, the UK, and other areas of the world were exposed to false information about US political figures spread across social media websites. It appears our ability to recognize pseudo-news of any sort may be challenging to some of us, as creating fake images and manipulating those images becomes more sophisticated. We need to be more critically attentive concerning the quality of journalism and the kind of media messages we're exposed to. We need to listen to our own inner guidance and our body's gut response as well, when we read information that doesn't resonate properly.

I spoke to a student well versed in journalism studies, and she voiced her concerns about the continued erosion of the quality and quantity of our local community-based news, news that provides core substance material and is integral to our national coverage.

It's important for high-quality, balanced, and credible journalism coverage to remain in place locally, regionally, and nationally. Balanced reporting is vital to let us know what is going on in the world, such as amazing innovations or contributions people are making in so many areas, accomplishments on behalf of the planet, people, and animals, lifesaving moments, healing miracles, stories of caring and kindness, and the way we support and help restore one another.

There is a simple solution: turn off the TV. If we can step back from this low-frequency energy programming and take a little more time to uplift ourselves through reading, taking up a hobby, walking out in nature, or developing an exercise routine, it can definitely help.

Positive activities might be considered a form of distraction, but they can also be a way to care about our minds and choose to allow positive information to influence us. Turning off the fear can help reduce some of our world's extreme news and other dramas that promote even more fear, stress, and anxiety through those specific portals.

Communication in Stressful Situations

We know stress, positive or negative, is part of life, but too much stress creates a constriction in our mind/body/spirit, and our vitality diminishes. As our energy is lowered, our perception of what is actually occurring around us also becomes more limited.

Again, we begin to default to the negative and develop tunnel vision, become judgmental, and make inaccurate assessments about the intentions and actions of others. We often don't hear what is actually being communicated, and we can misconstrue messages through an increasingly negative filter. Our communication can become less than hospitable, and we can start blaming others. Someone may be in a measure of distress, which may be showing up in them expressing their own irritation, and in that very moment, they may need us to be present to hear them, to bring a degree of patience and calmness to our listening, to recognize that they are actually feeling anxious or frightened and could benefit from receiving a caring response. We may not hear them if we ourselves are too stressed out and tense, and rather than mindfully responding to them, we may react by becoming annoyed ourselves, thus missing out on an opportunity to extend support, instead of adding more stress into the situation. You'll notice that when you are feeling more rested, coping with stress and other challenges becomes easier.

The Ease and Divisiveness of Gossip

Don Miguel Ruiz, author of the 1997 book *The Four Agreements: A Practical Guide to Personal Freedom*, emphasizes the power of the spoken word as a "gift from God," an essential tool in humanity's code of mindful conduct. With the right use of our words, we can either dishearten people or encourage them. We have the ability to use our words to help create healing situations and extend caring and compassion to each other. When we do this, we should know that our caring energy ripples out and extends beyond everyone we give support to.

People are naturally curious about each other; we like to positively share our own and others' interests, experiences, and accomplishments. However, there is a negative downside to our sharing: gossip.

Collins New English Dictionary (1999) defines *gossip* as "idle talk, usually about other people's private lives, especially of a disapproving or malicious nature." There is a difference between engaging in a natural, caring, and curious conversation and participating in unconsciously hostile gossip; this challenges our intention about the information we are sharing.

Gossip can often signal there are communication difficulties between friends, in our personal lives, or at work between colleagues or management and staff. There is often a fear or lack of skill about how to speak to one another safely and openly to resolve issues. Comments based on assumptions and perceptual distortions do not add to a positive tone in any relationship, and this happens more often when people experience excessive levels of stress and a lack of positive outlets. Here, our need to be mindful of our emotional states, our communication intentions, and our ways of managing our stress levels is important, especially if we notice our communications are veering off to the negative. More self-care in having additional downtime may be needed.

Gossip is actually very common in human communications, especially in the entertainment media. There is always a potential for misinformation. The following simple questions originating from Socrates can be helpful to consciously remind us of our intentions in our communication:

- Is it true?
- Is it kind?
- Is it necessary?

Our relationships can go more smoothly when we keep the intent of our communication as clear as possible and when we can react quickly if there are signs of tension, confusion, misinformation, or discord.

Vibrational Levels of Emotions

Throughout this chapter, we have explored many things that can affect our perceptions, our feelings, and our overall emotional states. We can actually fluctuate emotionally throughout our day with so many things we are now exposed to, with information coming at us from many directions. The stresses we experience from external sources, events, and incidents, combined with our own inner issues and feelings, can challenge our emotional state.

I will reiterate that we are emotionally sensitive people and need to appreciate that sensitivity as much as possible as we journey through our day. Recognizing what makes us feel down as well as what makes us feel happy, joyful, and peaceful brings us vital information in how we can better care for our minds, bodies, emotions, and spiritual natures. As we are vibrational beings, our feelings and emotional states have a vibration or frequency associated with them. We can feel negative or low, or we can feel more energized or higher or lighter.

In *Power vs. Force: The Hidden Determinations of Human Behaviour* (2012), David Hawkins explains how our emotional states can influence our vibrational frequencies and, ultimately, how we move from a higher vibrational energy to a much lower one. Having an ongoing sense of how we are feeling and what is affecting us is foundational to our self-care. We can operate in various kinds of emotional states, depending on which environment we are in at the time, who we are interacting with, how we feel physically, and many other interrelating factors. Hawkins describes an individual's overall level of consciousness as "the sum of the total effect of all these various levels" (97–98).

Hawkins's frequency levels show that when we are involved in feelings of shame, guilt, apathy, and grief, we are actually in such a low-energy level that it is similar to when we are entering a state of overall demise. When we are feeling fear, anger, desire, and pride, our vibrational level becomes more elevated from that lowered state. Finally, when we reach into the emotion of our inner courage, we allow for more life force to flow through us. We do feel better and far more energized. From that level of courage, we can move onward toward the most resilient and highest vibrational levels of love, joy, and enlightenment.

I relate to Hawkins's information to varying degrees, particularly in times of significant life losses. The amount of energy I've had in these times has been decisively lower as I moved through the grieving process. I felt mentally disrupted, my sleep was disturbed, I lacked an appetite, and I desired to become more isolated; my boundaries did not feel very strong, and my confidence was much lower. Grieving and loss states can have us feeling like we are moving through a dense fog or even physically like we are so low in our energy as to be almost walking through mud.

If we've ever had to work through any experiences of shame or guilt, in those times, our energy can plummet. Shame or guilt can be our response at times, if we have ever transgressed another's boundaries or felt we hurt someone. We may respond by feeling, *I am bad*, as is found in a low shame state, whereby we are more consumed by a lack of love for ourselves. In an emotional state of guilt, we haven't lost our core sense of self-regard, we have empathy for those we injured, and we feel bad about our actions and usually seek to remedy the situation.

As one can see from the levels below, the shame state is the lowest and slowest emotional and vibrational state. The following emotional vibrational states are condensed and extrapolated from Hawkins (Ibid., 97–116).

Level 20: Shame
Painful feeling of humiliation, distress, and whole person devaluing.

Level 30: Guilt
Feeling culpable for mistakes or offense in behavior; can also be a result of emotional manipulation.

Level 50: Apathy
Indifference, lack of concern, lethargy, passivity, unresponsive.

Level 75: Grief
Sorrow, dejection, despair, misery, anguish, deeply burdened.

Level 100: Fear
Fright, terror, agitation, alarm, anxiety, feeling under threat, immobilized.

Level 125: Desire
Wanting or wishing for something not received; can be experienced as a lacking.

Level 150: Anger
Annoyance, exasperation, hostility, indignation, irritability, and vengeance.

Level 175: Pride
A rise in self-esteem, but the ego is vulnerable to external opinions, which can fluctuate and send the vibration upward or downward to superiority.

Level 200: Courage
Strength or valor shown in the face of fear, terror, and grief.

Level 250: Neutrality
Ability to hold a peaceful, emotionally neutral observation.

Level 320: Willingness
Readiness to engage or assist in the moment; can be inspirational.

Level 350: Acceptance
Openly receiving a person or a situation as acceptable; expansion of perception.

Level 400: Reason
The ability to use the mind to integrate and present a wide variety of information for understanding with emotional objectivity.

Level 500: Love
A higher conscious experience of love as unconditional, void of attachment to outcomes, fear, or dependency on another. Loving above and through discord.

Level 540: Joy
Expansion of the unconditional aspect of love, such as patience and positivity. Notably hallmarked by compassion. A sense of lightness that arises from within, leading to inner joy and healing.

Level 600: Peace
A state that experiences transcendence, bliss, and self-realization; dissolution of religious affiliations; abiding awareness of the sacred energy or presence in all matter (aka God consciousness).

Level 700–1000: Enlightenment
The level of the nonduality and spiritually self-transcended divine masters or avatars in our history, such as Lord Krishna, Buddha, Lord Sananda, Swami Vivekanada, and Saint Germain, who mastered complete oneness and divine grace with all.

All of these levels, as they move from lower to highest vibrations, can help us appreciate our lack of energy when we have experienced emotional injury, are feeling down in the dumps, or are in a state of stress, fear, or anger. For many of us, these emotional states are situational and fluctuating. For others, they can remain static for longer periods of time.

Everyone's vibrational energy levels will fluctuate continuously and more acutely as unexpected changes occur and bring more uncertainty. In times of job loss, unexpected meetings with people not seen for years, or unexpected emotional ruptures with friends, family members, or colleagues, our emotional states can suddenly fluctuate as we attempt to discern and balance our feelings about what is occurring. Hawkins's emotional vibrational states are therefore worth keeping in mind as we look at what emotional energetic states lift or lower our energies.

As energy moves and is contagious, people in a family, a group of friends, or an organization can eventually impact the family, group, or organization as a whole, if they are routinely energizing to the positive or defaulting to the negative. On a personal level, it's important to recognize that change is continuously occurring, and how we cope and keep ourselves balanced is worth examining. This next section will look at some ways we can care for ourselves through changes.

Managing Changes

> *Everything we experience has a beginning, a middle and an end, and is followed by a new beginning. Therefore, do not draw back from the passage into darkness. When in deep water, become a diver.*
> —Ralph Blum (1987, 95)

Changes can bring uncertainty, self-doubt, fear, and an increased sense of vulnerability, even though we know changes are part of life. I have certainly had degrees of those feelings at various times when I've faced changes in my employment, housing, or relationships, as well as the death of loved ones. I've found, more often than not, that embracing or accepting changes, rather than denying or avoiding the changes and the feelings that arise, can make

Ultimate Self-Care

the kind of change more manageable because I'm not using as much of my energy in resisting it.

I generally don't mind change, as it gives me energy in its potential for new learning. Too much change, though, whether it be positive (such as receiving an exciting job offer, the birth of a baby, or bringing a new pet home) or negative (being laid off), can be more stressful and unpleasant if it occurs without a break, a period of transition. Changes occurring as a result of an emergency (e.g., accidents, severe weather, floods, fire) are more disruptive; traumatic events can certainly take much longer for adaptation, healing, and emotional balance to be restored.

Any of the aforementioned examples of changes in our lives can happen concurrently, of course, and though some of the changes might feel exciting, the experience can also be overwhelming. Depending on many personal factors, such as previous experience in dealing with changes, styles of coping with stress, available psychological and emotional supports, and present state of health, will have an impact on how well we manage change.

In *Managing Transitions: Making the Most of Change* (2009), author William Bridges writes about the impact of ongoing, accumulative changes: "We talk not of a single change but of change as an ongoing phenomenon. It is collage, not a simple image: one change overlaps with another, and it's all change as far as the eye can see" (99).

Bridges details the complexities and difficulties for people dealing with ongoing change; it isn't so much the pace of the change as the increased acceleration. As a result of not being able to acclimatize to the waves of change rushing in, we are thrown into perpetual transitions. He purports that each transition accompanying each level of change involves three phases, namely:

1. Where an ending, letting go, and losses of the old process are expressed.
2. A neutral zone, where there is a confused, in-limbo effect; an uncomfortable state of fluidity is felt, where new processes are not yet in place.
3. A new beginning with ambivalence, fears, complaints, or high fives; innovations are felt, with an eventual recognition to go forward (Ibid., 100–112).

These phases do not have clearly defined boundaries, and if there are multiple changes occurring at once, the overflowing cauldron of transitional shifts can stretch the most resilient person's ability to embrace change without suffering fatigue.

Currently, there seems to be changes under way across every spectrum in our world, as innovative opportunities are being created to advance us forward for our health and wellness, and environmental improvement projects and new ideas in resource management affect food sourcing and security. However, within the daily work world, many of these opportunities for change have increased, and employee stress levels have heightened; continuous change initiatives are under way, resulting in higher fatigue for workers. As Bridges mentions above, these changes may be occurring so swiftly and concurrently that they seem to be testing our personal and collective resilience. Below are some suggestions that can help us cope with changes on a more personal level.

Self-Care Strategies during Change

Paying attention to ourselves in how we are doing physically, emotionally, and psychologically is best as a regular routine for our self-care. As we have seen in a previous chapter, on a physical level, our body will tell us if we are experiencing unreleased levels of stress, and that includes stress brought on by seemingly smaller but continuous and accumulating stresses and changes (e.g., your car is in for a minor repair, and you're suddenly relying on public transit, resulting in inconvenient schedule changes, while at the same time, a family member is suddenly ill; you've also got a work meeting today that you're not ready for, and you have to get a root canal done, and your dog is going to have puppies any day).

Here are some important strategies for maintaining your self-care during changes:

- Pay attention to how your body feels and what your body needs in terms of good hydration, exercise, adequate sleep, and proper nutrition.
- Keep up as much of your regular routine, which also helps keep you grounded in times of change.
- Seek emotional and psychological support in sharing what you are experiencing during challenges, changes, and transitions.
- Stay connected with a supportive network of caring family, friends, or coworkers, or seek out a mental

health counselor who will keep you emotionally balanced.
- Practice the deep breathing and meditation exercises; this will also help keep you more grounded and clear-minded, to allow you to make better decisions.
- Maintain yourself in a quiet, relaxed atmosphere by turning off the TV and reading supportive books or articles; this will also help center and ground you, as will going out into nature.
- Make sure you keep listening to your inner self; intuitive nudges can help guide you during these challenging times, in allowing you to go with the flow or direct you to take action when it feels right.

A personal experience comes to mind when I needed to keep attending to my self-care, while I went through a significant time of change and loss.

Many years ago, I chose to leave a full-time job to focus on my Master of Social Work degree. I had completed only a portion of my studies and was looking for more work, as I was living on some limited funds for a time. In my employment pursuits, I wanted to ensure good self-care. That meant that I was prepared to turn down positions that would lead me to being stressed or burned out. These were not easy choices to make, as I generally enjoyed my work. However, I knew which jobs were going to be hard to manage, and I felt committed to my own health. My mother suddenly died during this time period, which shocked me (even though I'd had a premonition of this event), and I felt vulnerable in dealing with my grief.

Ultimate Self-Care

Shortly after her death, I realized I had miscalculated the income I had at my disposal, which meant my rent payment was in jeopardy. I felt very anxious and sent up a prayer to be guided to resolve this situation. I decided I needed to try and relax and stay grounded so I could think more clearly. I decided to go for a long run.

Feeling calmer afterward, a thought suddenly entered my mind: I was near a previous work site and decided to drop in to say hello to the director. Susan, who was rarely in her office, just happened to be free and asked me if I'd seen the part-time coordinator position posted on their board. I was surprised because in my intense job search, I had not spotted this posting anywhere. Although it was low pay, I applied and was grateful when I was hired. I didn't recognize it at the time, but given my state of exhaustion and vulnerability from everything surrounding my mother's recent death, and still needing to go on with my studies, this job was actually the perfect transitional position for me. It helped support me financially and emotionally until I regained my inner strength and self-confidence to move forward with more energy.

In retrospect, I can see that paying attention to my self-care first, in regaining some physical and emotional grounding and calmness, allowed me to listen to my intuition, which signaled to me to make that fateful connection with the director, at that specific time. It all played a part in gently guiding me to what I truly needed during that difficult time of transition.

Barbara Halcrow, MSW

Self-Care as Family Caregivers

In the previous section, I mentioned that as a social worker, I wanted to be more vigilant in maintaining my health in order to avoid fatigue and burnout. Several decades working in social services and health care has allowed me to see that many of these roles lead to the symptoms of mental, emotional, and physical fatigue, sometimes termed "compassion fatigue," which has been a concern for almost all of us in the people-helping fields.

The Collins New English Dictionary (1999, 150) defines *compassion fatigue* as "the inability to react sympathetically to a disaster because of over-exposure to previous disasters." Compassion fatigue is most easily understood if we consider that dealing with intense, upsetting, and sometimes traumatic situations on a frequent basis, without stepping away to rest and rejuvenate ourselves, drains us emotionally, mentally, and physically; we are not able to fully feel our compassion for others. This means we are not present within ourselves and risk not being mentally or emotionally present and aware for those we are giving care to.

Compassion fatigue symptoms include the following:

- emotional and mental exhaustion
- diminished ability to feel empathy or compassion
- insensitivity
- reduced enjoyment of previous activities
- lack of clarity in decision making

Ultimate Self-Care

- irritability, anger, and rage
- hypersensitivity or insensitivity to emotional material
- susceptibility to illness

(F. Mathieu, *Running on Empty: Compassion Fatigue in Health Professionals,* 2007)
http://www.compassionfatigue.org/pages/RunningOnEmpty.pdf

If extensive fatigue sets in, we may not recognize it; we can make mistakes in giving care, such as giving the wrong medications, being too exhausted to perform some duties, losing patience with the person in our care, not recognizing when she or he needs emergency intervention. In short, we can become increasingly insensitive, detached, and unaware of how neglectful we are becoming of ourselves and the very people we are giving care to.

Compassion fatigue is also a concern for those who are giving care to a family member. Family caregivers can be adult children, parents, spouses, or even a close family friend who are providing physical or emotional care at home to an elderly or disabled loved one. These duties can include assisting with personal care (bathing, dressing, feeding), giving medications, and more.

Being a family caregiver can be a new role that happens due to a sudden accident, an injury from war, or an elderly family member who is in decline.

Even if we want to care for a loved one at home, this role can bring a greater challenge to look after ourselves. We are often less likely to offer the same commitment to provide care for ourselves. I have seen that caregivers tend to sacrifice even more of their personal time and energy when it comes to their family members. Some may not ask for additional help in feeling they should be able to handle everything.

They may have greater difficulty letting anyone else care for their family member, believing they offer a special, more personal form of care they know their loved one really prefers. In our desire to care perfectly and lovingly, our own needs can become secondary. We might well find our ability to say no to increasing demands of caregiving becomes weaker, and we can become extremely worn out. Compassion fatigue and its exhaustive elements will gain on us.

As previously mentioned, if we work in social services, health care, or any people-helping occupations, we need to be vigilant about our self-care to prevent cumulative exhaustion. If we are also caring for a loved one, we can find ourselves on a fast track to stress-related illnesses and compassion fatigue when performing dual roles, essentially burning the candle at both ends. Whatever your role, it's important to pay attention to your own needs and assess how you are feeling. If you are a family caregiver, check out your regional health care agencies or local health units to inquire about any specific supports offered for family caregivers.

Teva Canada Caregivers (https://tevacaregivers.com) and Family Care Giving Alliance (https://www.caregiver.org/caregiving) are two comprehensive support networks with resources for Canada and the United States, respectively.

In the next chapter, we will examine how we can further help ourselves when we are at work or at home by exploring and strengthening our personal and collective resilience.

CHAPTER 6

BUILDING OUR RESILIENCE

While we covered a wide range of topics related to self-care in previous chapters, this chapter will focus more on caring for our physical well-being.

Resilience

Resilience is part of our own inner self-care and self-sustaining mechanism. It's how we bounce back from difficult experiences. It is the process of adapting well in the face of adversity, trauma, tragedy, threats, or even significant sources of stress, such as family and relationship problems, serious health issues, workplace difficulties, and financial stressors. It shows us the strength of our spirit in the face of powerful odds.

Research has shown that resilience is a routine response for most of us. It involves behaviors, thoughts, and actions that can be learned and developed (American Psychological Association 2016). That's good news because we can then strengthen what already exists.

We know that our resilience begins when our body is forming our earliest neuro coding for our cognitive functions. This coding comes at a time when we begin interacting with our outer environment and understanding what's needed for survival.

Barbara Halcrow, MSW

Resilience then grows to encompass a dual understanding of what we feel we need to achieve for a sense of happiness within us, as well as how we are able to use the resources around us. We need to survive, and we also want to thrive.

Outer Resilience Resources

Our Primary Relationships

One of the primary factors contributing to resilience is our ability to form nourishing, loving relationships. Relationship building begins with our family relationships, especially with our parents and siblings. These relationships impart a powerful and lifelong imprint for each of us. They are critical in our experience of being supported and are where trust building, belonging, and behavior modelling occurs. Maintaining positive relationships with supportive family, friends, and colleagues is perhaps the most important resilience element of all.

Our Spiritual, Cultural, or Community Support

When change comes into our lives, we cope best with a sense of community. Connecting with supportive people who share a circle of support with a common bond is vital in our resilience to withstand changes. This sharing and mirroring help keep things in perspective and gently remind us of our essential belongingness, sacredness, and worthiness in the world. This important support can also strengthen our inner resilience reserves, described below.

Inner Resilience Resources

Acknowledge Our Strengths

The ability to have insight into our own strengths is essential. It helps us to keep a positive perspective and have confidence in ourselves, no matter the circumstances. We saw earlier that there is a human tendency to default to the negative, and we can counteract this by consciously affirming our strengths and skills.

Accomplish Realistic Goals

It can be easier to set short-term, even daily, and longer-term goals that can be successfully reached in realistic time frames. It's good to remain committed to our goals but also flexible to make any needed adjustments. If we start with the smaller, easier goals that we know we can accomplish, we can build upon each achievement and congratulate ourselves.

Focus on Solving Problems

Solution-focused problem solving is the ability to appreciate what is actively working in our lives and what our strengths are, instead of focusing on our deficits. In this way, we look at what we want rather than what we don't want. This way of problem solving examines any exceptions as to when the problem is not occurring and seeing if we can use those exceptions to work toward our solutions in a different way (Priest and Gass 1997).

Emotional Self-Management

Emotional self-management is our ability to recognize the full range of our feelings and emotions, and manage them effectively. This learning can include strengthening ourselves emotionally, particularly in those situations that trigger our anger and any tendency to blame. Emotional self-management gives us more emotional intelligence in trusting ourselves to manage any situation. The overall result is a boost in our self-esteem and confidence.

Broader Resilience Resources

Cultural Competency

An important strategy for building resiliency is cultivating cultural competency to foster our greater community. When we are open to each other's different perspectives and understand our cultural differences and similarities, the bonds we create can strengthen our knowledge, acceptance, and sense of what community really can mean. Cultural competency involves learning about the specific behaviors, attitudes, and spiritual practices of those we live and work with. By being genuinely interested in knowing about others, we show respect for their culture and enhance interactions in our diverse communities. When we embrace openness and seek to become culturally competent, we build more strength and significantly increase the sense of global unity.

In viewing how people practice self-care in times of significant change, it's essential to appreciate that individuals react in different ways to traumatic events or stresses. There can be striking differences in people's perceptions and their ability to reach out for help or discuss their experiences. Overall, I have found that families in larger communities can be quite cohesive in maintaining their degrees of inner strength and support of their loved ones. For example, I have given support to friends from Indo-Canadian, Chinese, Jewish, Japanese, Italian, and First Nations cultures whose loved ones have died; I always ask in advance about proper protocol for dress and behavior. There are variations in how inclusive some cultures are in having others participate in ceremonies for the deceased. There are differences in how the families and close friends of the bereaved display their grief, perform funeral rituals, and spiritually care for the deceased in the afterlife.

Developing cultural competency needs to be ongoing, as we need to appreciate that people also leave their homes with little or no preparation to enter a new cultural experience.

LGBTQ2S Communities

Cultural competency also involves understanding and honoring Lesbian, Gay, Bisexual, Transgendered, Queer, and Two-Spirited (LGBTQ2S) community members. Canada recognizes and respects the rights and freedoms of the LGBTQ2S peoples and continues to openly celebrate these communities with yearly Pride parades. But in too many other countries, individuals are still being denied recognition, inclusion, and respect. Many of our LGBTQ2S peoples have been exiled from their own religious, spiritual, or community cultures of origin. Many have chosen to leave for their own mental, spiritual, and physical wellness and safety.

Inclusive acceptance of sexual orientation and gender identity is still being battled in real life-and-death situations; in some countries, homophobia remains pervasively alive in its many forms. There is a profound lack of knowledge in the world regarding the breadth and beauty of the expression of our human sexuality, which I believe is also connected to the vitality of the human spirit.

My feeling is that this fear about our true loving natures, expressed in sexual intimacy, will take a longer time to be eradicated, for our human wholeness to find its way into full acceptance worldwide. Individually, we should offer ourselves and one another love and acceptance, combined with human sexuality education and legislative changes on behalf of the LGBTQ2S peoples across the globe; these implementations will help erode centuries of ignorance, fear, and oppression and move all of humanity toward understanding, equality, and freedom.

Nutrition in Self-Care

Good nutrition is a cornerstone of optimal health. Many of us have our own cultural preferences in our relationship with food, as it can hold spiritual symbolism and meaning for our health and wellness.

In some spiritual practices, like Ayurveda, our body is a sacred temple. What we place in it needs to do more than nourish our body; it must also honor and support our higher spiritual being that is ultimately connected to the divine, and it is an important acknowledgment of our need to be mindful in our eating.

This mindfulness is necessary because, as food is alive with its own life force, it makes sense to choose more natural foods over packaged and processed foods, which has far less energy to nourish our bodies.

In British Columbia, First Nations peoples are culturally connected to the land, water, fish, wildlife, and plant life. Food holds traditional spiritual meaning; we need to preserve and protect the environment and its inhabitants. Traditional harvesting of animals, fish, and plants for maximum nutritional benefits is carried out with mindfulness of the need for self-sufficiency and the preservation and conservation of life.

"Go to the land and waters to find your first foods. Be active in exercising your right to hunt, fish, harvest, and gather in your territory. Ask the old people and the traditional and environmental knowledge keepers how to do this in a good way. It will be good for the mind, body, and spirit and contribute to a self-reliant future" (First Nations Health Authority 2016).

What Should I Eat?

For many of us, our relationship with food can be complex and even confusing at times. There seems to be so much misinformation as to what we should and should not be eating for our best health. We have developed dietary issues like diabetes and celiac disease, and we need to consider whether to eat gluten-free or not. Some of us are looking at our potential allergies to food, and we have concerns regarding genetically modified organisms (GMOs), questionable food additives, and their impact on our digestive system. There has been an overall degradation of the quality of our food, and we are encouraged to use health food supplements to make up that difference.

Dr. Vandana Shiva, author, activist, and scientific advisor, has researched and lectured globally on the nature and direction of the world's changes occurring in our food and nutritional resources, as well as the concerns involving GMO foods. Shiva (2014) cites the urgent need to return to the rich diversity we once had; there used to be eighty-five hundred species of foods that provided our body with optimal nutritional health.

There is an increase in the belief that there is more nutritious bang for your buck when eating whole, organic, and grass-fed foods. However, there is an unfortunate increase in cost involved, making these nourishing foods more expensive. People living on low incomes often must choose lower cost, high sugar, fatty, and carbohydrate-rich foods to survive. We know in healing and health care services that good nutrition is strongly encouraged for disease prevention. Type 2 diabetes, for example, has been linked to poverty.

The energy related to the quality of food and nutrition affects every cell of our brain and body, helping to preserve our mental recall, learning, physical responses, and emotional stasis. Emotionally, food also becomes a means of coping when stress levels rise. We often go for quick comfort, and too often, sugar is one of the most available substances to quell the stress response.

Andrew Weil, author of *Spontaneous Healing* (1995), says that our diet is a significant part of maintaining our longevity; he adds, "Fortunately, or unfortunately, we live in a world that tempts us with a great variety and abundance of food, and many of us eat not to satisfy hunger but to ally anxiety, depression, and boredom, to provide a substitute for emotional nourishment, or to try to fill an inner void" (170).

When I initially worked closely with people with mental health and addictions, the pervasive negative impact of sugar became quickly apparent. Like the opioids morphine and heroin, sugar has a similar effect on certain pathways of the brain, which results in a sense of craving for more of the substance when its ingestion is followed by cessation.

Over time, our ability to regulate that substance is diminished, and we need more of it to get the same dopamine pleasure effect to calm us. Our ability to resist the temptation of sugary substances in junk food ends up not being about a lack of willpower but about the development of our brain's and body's response, a response that resembles that of a drug addict. It's no small wonder so many of us have eating disorders.

Moving toward healthier eating habits takes time. It takes gentle patience to learn about the role of food in our lives and how we can become aware of what we are eating, what it is and is not giving us, and why we are drawn to certain foods and substances. In *Super Brain* (2012), Chopra and Tanzi examine the issue of disordered eating on the spectrum from anorexia to obesity. They say that in order to help ourselves come back into a balanced state, we need to rebalance our brain; it's the key to the solution.

Barbara Halcrow, MSW

"The key is to bring our brain into balance, then use its ability to balance everything—hormones, hunger, cravings, and habits. Your weight is all in your head because, ultimately, your body is in your head. That is, the brain lies at the source of all bodily functions, and your mind lies at the source of your brain" (97).

The authors claim that if an eating imbalance occurs, accommodating that imbalance by continuing to adapt or work around our weight problem creates even a greater imbalance. They make this argument because "imbalance feeds more imbalance," and it becomes a truly vicious circle, ultimately resulting in grave health consequences (Ibid., 98). Chopra and Tanzi suggest that the brain has the capacity to rectify physical imbalances; in that regard, they urge readers to

- stop fighting with yourself,
- give up diet foods,
- ignore calorie counting, and
- work to restore balance in areas that create imbalance: stress, emotions, and sleep.

Again, this is where we need to consciously try to make time to find out what is going on within ourselves. What are our stress trigger points? Are there any areas of unresolved emotional issues? This is a time when we need to become gentle and compassionate observers. When we recognize a change is needed, though, it is time to take action on our own behalf.

Detoxification

People participate in detoxification processes for a variety of reasons. Some people want to abstain for a period of time from all forms of sugar, wheat, dairy, or another food group. Some people find it necessary to lose extra weight for improved fitness and appearance. Withdrawing from certain food groups sometimes results in the increase in other food categories and methods of preparation (e.g., juicing) or with the addition of specific herbs to promote toxins to be released.

Detoxifying the body can reveal much information concerning potential allergies and other manifestations of physical irritants and ailments during or after a detoxification process. I feel any form of detoxification must be done gently and thoughtfully and usually in consultation with a health practitioner, as mentioned below.

The overall benefits of some forms of food withdrawal can include weight loss, clearer thinking, increased energy, stronger immunity, clearer skin, shinier hair, improved sleep patterns, hormonal balancing, and decreased muscle or joint pain, to name a few.

There are many forms of detoxifications that can last for several days, weeks, or even as a regular lifestyle shift, depending on your specific goals and your health. I am aware of people who have gone on strict water fasts or juice fasts for several days to several weeks and reported a notable increase in their vitality and even significant spiritual insights. These fasts have not suited me up to this point in my life. However, I have found great benefit in detoxifying my body to physically, emotionally, and psychologically clear away my attachment to sugar, simple carbohydrates, and wheat, for example. I usually do this dietary withdrawal several times a year, for at least two weeks at a time. For me, as for many of us, I am sugar sensitive, and sugar is contained in far too many foods. Restricting as much sugar and wheat as possible has proven to be one of the best diet alterations I can make.

As our needs and our bodies change over time, it can be confusing to figure out what kind of detoxification process is best, and therefore, it is important to research any plan and consult fully with your physician or health care consultant.

Additional information and support for our nutritional needs can also come from a local community health center's dietitian, a holistic nutritionist, a naturopath, or a support group, if we feel we are somewhere on the continuum of disordered eating. We may need to get specific organ, gland, blood, or hormonal tests (sometimes through saliva) to find out more details about how we are functioning and what we need if we are out of balance or in nutritional deficiency.

Herbs and Spices

Herbs and spices are an area of invaluable information and assistance to our health care. Herbs and spices offer significant rewards for mind and body functions, immune boosting, healing, and detoxification, and they are a contributing factor in overall healthy living and aging.

Globally, the ancients and Aboriginal peoples were the first herbalists in their use of thousands of plants, shrubs, and trees, with specific rituals to purify and heal the mind, body, and spirit. We routinely benefit from the use of

Echinacea, goldenseal, ginseng, gotu kola, garlic, ginger, lavender, pepper, cloves, nutmeg, turmeric, and chilies, to name but a fraction of helpful herbs and spices (Mindell 1992).

Many communities have skilled herbalists and naturopaths who have studied the work passed on over centuries and provide us with this beneficial information to improve our health and wellness. I have decisively benefited by being guided by herbalists and naturopaths; although we have many fine physicians in our communities, I have found that few are educated about the nutritional needs of clients. There are also community and online courses for learning the role of specific food groups, their impact, and how we can keep ourselves functioning optimally. [13]

Additionally, more information on First Nations medicine is noted below.[14]

The Vibrational Color of Food

There's a reason your parents said, "Eat your greens." Food also has an energetic vibration, and its color is certainly

---

[13] David "Avocado" Wolfe's online Living Nutrition e-course through the BodyMind Institute is very information, interesting, and easy to follow (https://shop.davidwolfe.com/products/david-avocado-wolfe-living-nutrition-e-course)

[14] Further information on First Nations medicine can be found at Anthony J. Cichoke, *Secrets of Native American Herbal Remedies: A Comprehensive Guide to the Native American Tradition of Using Herbs and the Mind/Body/Spirit Connection for Improving Health and Well-Being* (New York: Penguin Publishers, 2001); Turtle Island Native Network: *Healing and Wellness,* http://www.turtleisland.org/healing/healing-wellness.htm

an aspect of how food affects our body's energy systems. Specifically, the various colors of different foods indicate they contain specific kinds of antioxidants and other kinds of nutrients that act to maintain our body's health.[13] For example:

Green foods: broccoli, asparagus, olives, avocado, pears, limes, and green grapes offer support and blood purification.

Red foods: red apples, tomatoes, and strawberries offer antioxidants and beta-carotene to neutralize free radicals.

Orange foods: carrots, squash, sweet potatoes, oranges, apricots, melons, egg yolk, turmeric, and ginger also provide minerals, antioxidants, and vitamin C.

Yellow foods: yellow peppers, parsnips, yams, grapefruit, lemons, pineapples, and pears offer more sun-derived antioxidants, plus iron, magnesium, zinc, and vitamins B and E.

Blue foods: seaweed, asparagus, plums, blueberries, and boysenberries are rich in vital minerals and antioxidants.

Purple foods: eggplant, plums, purple grapes, blackberries, and lavender help to calm nervous system disorders.

Some foods have several colors associated with them because they change color when cooked.

Aside from the various authors and other resources we can access, we need to structure a healthy food plan that works for each of us, given our lifestyles, our preferences, our coping methods, our income, and the kind of supports around us. Goodreads[15] has a comprehensive list of

---

[15] https://www.goodreads.com/list/show/7183.A_Nutrition_Reading_List

recommended nutritional books to choose from to help guide you.

Blessing Our Food

Blessing food, as in saying grace, may seem unnecessary or old-fashioned, unless you are in keeping with a faith that maintains the practice of saying a blessing or prayer before eating. Actually, blessing food increases the vibration of the food we eat. When we send positive regard or simple appreciation for our food, it absorbs the positive energy we send to it, and that also helps nourish our bodies better.

As often as one can remember, it is good to at least give inner gratitude to your food and ask that the food provide you with maximum nourishment. It's a simple thing to do, but it allows a sense of increased gratitude to become part of our eating habits.

An example of a simple blessing is, "We offer gratitude for this food and may this food be blessed with love and provide us with all the nourishment we need."

Water

Along with caring that the food we eat provides us with good nutrition for our wellness, we should also be concerned about the quantity and quality of the water available to us. As we are primarily composed of water, it's important to ensure we are adequately hydrated with filtered, non-fluoridated water throughout the day. Sometimes, instead of feeling hungry, we are really feeling thirsty.

Brenda Watson (2008, 141) suggests that we drink half our body weight in ounces of water per day. For example, a 140-pound person would drink 70 ounces. Drinking more water gives us a number of positive health benefits:

- It increases metabolism and energy.
- It acts as natural daily detoxification.
- When adding lemon juice or apple cider vinegar to water, it helps alkalize the body, increases bile, and flushes out the kidneys.
- It helps prevent constipation.
- It improves skin tone.

Water Quality

Where I live, our watershed has no added fluoridated water (http://yourwatermatters.com/vancouver-water/top-11questions-about-metro-vancouver-tap-water/).

There still continues to be an ongoing debate on the efficacy of fluoridation in water to protect and strengthen tooth enamel against acid erosion, plaque, and bacteria.[14] Many Canadian dental associations still encourage the use of fluoride.

The Canadian Dental Association (cdc.adc.ca) also supports the use of fluoride being added to water, "to protect all members of the community from tooth decay. Community water fluoridation is a safe and effective way of preventing tooth decay at a low cost."

However, another study shows that fluoride actually has a significant calcification effect on the pineal gland because "fluoride accumulates easily in the brain" (Luke 2001, par. 11).

Further, a report from the National Research Council found that "fluoride is likely to cause decreased melatonin production and to have other effects on normal pineal function, which in turn could contribute to a variety of effects in humans" (2007, 256).

As mentioned in chapter 1, the pineal gland is associated with one of the seven powerful chakras in our body and is sometimes called the "seat of the soul." It is associated with our brain's functions. Researchers for some years have expressed concern regarding the connection of sodium fluoride's impact on the pineal gland with the development of cognitive diminishment, decreased insight, and even Alzheimer's disease.

Obviously, this can be a complex issue, with benefits to enamel protection, as proposed by the dental industry, while other scientific examinations present opposing views, in terms of the accumulative effects of absorbing varying amounts of fluoride. If one is concerned enough to want to explore recovery from any degree of decalcification of the pineal gland and add more health into one's diet, it might be best to consult your own dentist, as well as a naturopathic doctor, a nutritionist, or a health food consultant. Allow for your own conclusions and listen to your body's responses to the information to give you clues as to what feels right. Additionally, some foods assist in whole body wellness by decalcifying the pineal gland, such as walnuts, neem extract, spirulina, apple cider vinegar, coconut oil, turmeric, and ginger. There are further articles of interest concerning the fluoride concerns noted in the footnote.[16]

By focusing on areas of nutrition, hydration, coping, and stress reduction, we can do well along our nutritional path, but we may become undermined by another critical part of our self-care: getting adequate sleep.

The Importance of Sleep

"How are you this morning?"
"Not bad, just a little sleep deprived."

Adequate sleep is critical; the body continually needs to repair tissue and for all-around restorative health. Each of us has an internal circadian rhythm, a twenty-four-hour body clock that is affected by sunlight, temperature, our behavior, and our lifestyle. This master clock also controls the production of the hormone melatonin, significant for a good night's sleep (National Institute of General Medical Sciences 2016).

The literature on sleep shows people differ in terms of how many hours of sleep we need to function well, according

---

[16] "Should Canadian Communities Continue to Fluoridate Water?" (https://healthydebate.ca/2015/07/topic/evidence-for-fluoridated-water); "The Fluoride Debate", CBC Archives (https://www.cbc.ca/archives/topic/the-fluoride-debate; "Pineal Gland" from Wikipedia (https://en.wikipedia.org/wiki/Pineal_gland).
C. R. Bayliss, N. L. Bishop, and R. C. Fowler. "Pineal Gland Calcification and the Defective Sense of Direction." *British Medical Journal* 291, 21–28, December 1985. (https://www.ncbi.nlm.nih.gov/pmc/articles/PMC1419179/).

to our age, lifestyle, work routines, physical activity, stress, depression, and anxiety issues; the particular life stage we are in may result in hormonal fluctuations.

According to *The Canadian Sleep Review Current Issues, Attitudes and Advice to Canadians* (2016), "Many Canadians are functioning with chronic sleep debt, a pervasive issue and a significant health concern for many people, affecting many segments of the population."

The Mayo Clinic reports that a consistent lack of sleep – less than five hours for men and less than six hours for women – is also a factor in weight gain. A natural response to lack of sleep is to reduce activity. A lack of sleep response is also to increase food and other sugar substances to boost energy levels. This response is because sleep affects ghrelin and leptin, hormones associated with regulating the appetite (Hensrud 2015).

The Canadian Sleep Review (2016) also claims that Canadians do not give sleep their highest priority, yet we are quite knowledgeable about the dos and don'ts when planning on getting a good sleep. Specific sleep disruptions are related to relationship discord, willingness to sacrifice sleep to fit in other activities, work or home life stresses, inability to adapt to ongoing home and work changes, long distances commuting between work and home, excessive exposure to computer screens, working more than one job, illness, change of diet, and hormonal changes. All these areas adversely affect sleep, and in turn, the lack of sleep contributes to significant performance problems and health and safety issues.

"An alarming 20 percent of Canadians admit to falling asleep at the wheel at least once over the last year. Studies also suggest fatigue is a factor in about 15 percent of motor vehicle collisions, resulting in about 400 deaths and 2,100 serious injuries every year" (Canada Safety Council 2009).

Insomnia

The Canadian Sleep Society describes insomnia as an inability to sleep properly and specifically involves sleep patterns such as difficulty falling asleep, waking up in the middle of the night and not being able to fall back asleep, poor quality of sleep if sleeping too lightly, and waking up too early in the morning and not getting back to sleep. Chronic sleep deprivation can be a singular contributing source of depression (Morin 2014).

The society addresses insomnia and sleep issues that primarily stem from anxiety, depression, and stress, but can also include chronic pain and side effects from the use of over-the-counter medication.

Insomnia can occur when we are in transition of any kind, as our inner energies will shift and change. This occurs when someone or an animal close to us dies, we move to a new home, or we change jobs.

Sudden sleep changes can also occur with transitions connected to emotional and spiritual insights. These insights can happen when we go through intense therapy to resolve traumas or step away from addictions. It can also happen when we are touched by an event or a situation that triggers these deeper insights and opens up our energy system, meaning any one of our chakras can become more open, allowing increased energy to run through us.

Ultimate Self-Care

These openings can be subtle or dramatic, but opening to new insights, feelings, or long-forgotten memories can be an aspect of our spiritual growth. As more energy is released, we can better open our spiritual senses. These experiences, although positive, can also be painful when we let go. They can be disruptive and throw us off our normal routine.

The disruptions do calm down after a while when our minds, emotions, and physical bodies begin to catch up to the spiritual growth that's occurring. We can rebalance, but we still need to try and make personal and environmental adjustments to cope. We also need to ask for the right help. If we are suffering from any form of insomnia and aren't sure what the underlying cause is, or if we have been physically injured or traumatized in any way, and sleep issues are hampering our health and recovery, we should seek help from a physician or mental health counselor. There are various avenues to improve sleep, including prescription medication (short-term only, as drug dependency is real and dangerous), behavior therapy, and herbal supplements, which are not regulated. Before spending money on prescriptions or other supplements, the following suggestions may help.

Suggestions for Improved Sleep

First, we need to prioritize sleep. We need to see it as paramount in our daily plan for good self-care and make changes to get the required sleep we need. Sleep deprivation over time becomes too costly to our mental, emotional, and physical functioning. Ensure your bedroom is as dark, quiet, and comfortable as possible. Black-out curtains that are heat insulated are most effective in keep your room dark. Using soft-ear plugs and wearing a sleep mask can also assist in creating a darker, quieter atmosphere. Some people play CDs that have soft water or nature sounds that can create a white noise for a soothing atmosphere.

Here are some other suggestions:

- Avoid all stimulants like caffeine or nicotine a few hours before bedtime, as well as sugar substances, including alcohol, to avoid sleep disruptions.
- Avoid watching TV news late in the evening, as it tends to increase anxiety and stress, and we're more vulnerable to its impact at bedtime.
- If it feels right for you physically, exercise later on in the day; it can help relax you for the evening.
- Many find it beneficial to journal your concerns of the day to avoid ruminating on them later on.
- Reading before going to bed to divert attention from the day can be effective in creating calmness, but avoid lengthy reading on computer screens and tablets, as the type of light they emanate stimulates your system.
- Consider eating a low-carb snack before bedtime to mitigate a drop in your blood sugar, which can result in wakefulness during the night.
- If you can meditate or deep breathe at bedtime and focus solely on your breath, you might find this practice highly effective in bringing calm. Some people find it helpful to count down from 20 while focusing their mind on their breath.

- Work toward getting up at the same time every morning, if possible, to help your body become more regulated. Drinking herbal tea at bedtime (like Sleepy Time or chamomile tea) can calm you and encourage sleep. Health food stores carry a wide variety of teas, or you might choose to consult with an herbalist or holistic health consultant.

Try using a sleep application such as mysleepbutton.com. This application was recently developed by a Simon Fraser University professor, Dr. Luc Beaudoin, and has already shown considerable promise for those suffering from sleep difficulties. This app also garnered the interest of Oprah Winfrey and was showcased on *Global News*, May 3, 2017 (http://globalnews.ca/news/3423143/b-cprofessors-sleep-technique-gets-attention-from-oprah/).

Changes to increase your hours of sleep can take time and test your patience. Again, it's good to consult with your physician, a counselor, psychologist, or a trusted friend to share and get more information to reduce anxiety, stress, grief, or depression. It's too uncomfortable and emotionally painful to suffer through nights of sleep deprivation and not seek help.

Physical Exercise

The topic of exercise covers a large amount of information, but it's certainly a vital one to keep our bodies working optimally. How much, how often, when to work out, and what form of exercise to sustain one's self-care varies as to each individual's state of health, physical build and capability, interest, lifestyle, and specific goals.

I have spent my life participating in all kinds of activities for enjoyment and used my energy to ensure a balanced lifestyle and manage the stresses that occurred. Health and exercise regimes change over time. At this time in my life, I try to ensure a daily walking or cycling routine, with strength maintenance exercises three days a week at the gym.

Given the vastness of the subject, I suggest that each of us start what is simple and reasonable and what we already know of ourselves. Start any new routine with what is easiest and build from there. Buddy up with someone who has similar goals to encourage each other.

The John Hopkins Medical online health website (2019) encourages involvement in aerobics, strength training, core exercises, balance training, flexibility, and stretching as the most essential forms of exercise to keep us healthy and fit at any age (https://www.hopkinsmedicine.org/health/wellness-and-prevention/3-kinds-of-exercise-that-boost-heart-health).

This information is corroborated by the Harvard Medical School's *Harvard Health,* which describes the five best exercises for ongoing health and fitness, particularly if you are not into an intense regime of exercise but do want to keep fit as you mature: swimming, tai chi, strength training, walking, and Kegel exercises (https://www.health.harvard.edu/staying-healthy/5-of-the-best-exercises-you-can-ever-do).

If you are concerned about any ongoing health issues, it is always wise to consult with your family physician before you begin a new physical regime, in order to make safest choices for any current physical, emotional, or mental challenges you are working with.

This chapter has taken us through some areas that explore how we can increase our resilience by how we connect in our personal and community relationships and appreciate the richness of the various interconnecting, diverse cultures that interweave with our lives. We also looked more closely at what ways we increase our overall physical health and wellness self-care practices.

Getting through difficult times that create upheavals can also involve going deeper within ourselves to bring forward more of our inner wisdom. If we make more time to spend with ourselves, through a simple meditation, just lying down for a few minutes, or walking outside in a quiet environment, it can help clear, quiet, and ground you. The next chapter will look at ways to strengthen our inner reserves: the deeper feeling realms, connected to our mental health and spiritual aspects of our self-care.

CHAPTER 7

INCREASING STRENGTH THROUGH INNER DOORS

Compassion is strength.

There are times where we just want to be alone and quiet with ourselves in deeper reflection to get to know ourselves better, or to just take a timeout from daily stresses. Taking time away might seem almost impossible if we are feeling completely stretched for time with a lot of responsibilities related to our job, family, or community involvement.

If we are actually able to take time for contemplation, and re-energizing, beginning with short time frames of a few minutes to a few hours here and there, we can gradually extend it to longer time frames to make it really worthwhile. More relaxed quiet time brings an increase in our awareness, objectivity, and problem solving, while it refreshes our senses. Making time for ourselves allows us to see if we are really taking our lives forward in the direction we want or if we need to make some changes.

I have a friend who, in past years, would spend months on top of a forest fire lookout in the Yukon Territory. These were incredibly solitary times for her, but she told me they were also times of personal deepening and connecting to nature and what her own spirituality held for her.

Barbara Halcrow, MSW

Communing at length with our natural surroundings is to me one of the best forms of solace and retreat.

People who spend significant time in various kinds of retreats often find they've returned with a significantly changed view of life, of their relationships, and themselves. I certainly have practiced taking vacation weeks as forms of needed change and retreat into restful solitude and learning and meditation, especially in nature, and also greatly enjoy stepping out of retreat mode to meet new people in different environments.

There are many ways to go about finding our own inner revelations in places of rest and rejuvenation. The following information and suggestions were helpful to others and to me. Since we hold many answers to life's hurdles inside ourselves, if we dedicate enough time and space, we can practice accessing those insights much more easily and strengthen our confidence and self-reliance in the process. These are some vital areas to consider when we want to see our lives unfold more peacefully. It starts inside of us.

Every Feeling Counts

> *To ignore, repress, or dismiss our feelings*
> *is to fail to listen to the stirrings of the Spirit*
> *within our emotional life.*
> —Brennan Manning

One of the most difficult things we do in our lifetime is learning to accept all of our feelings, even the gnarliest ones. In Western culture, we still tend toward a more conservative or stoic style of not showing our feelings, especially with feelings of grief, hurt, sadness, fear, guilt, or embarrassment. If we do express some of these feelings, there can be a lingering concern of whether we are expressing our feelings appropriately or if we risk being considered too sensitive, too emotional, too this, or too that.

Generally, most people seem to avoid the overall experience of feeling awkward and vulnerable when experiencing or expressing their feelings. Vulnerability has had many public commentaries in recent years to bring to light that there is strength in showing our lovingness, tenderness, anxiety, shyness, awkwardness, uncertainty, confusion, and other feelings that might make us fear being unprotected, and at risk of being hurt or diminished in some way. To live our lives to the fullest in the breadth and richness of our own humanity means taking risks in moving beyond our emotional fears and risking appearing weak, soft, foolish, uninformed, unintelligent, or simply not part of the group.

Our feelings are integrally connected to all our energy systems, as shown in previous chapters, and they have a decisive impact on all parts of our functioning. If we choose to open as fully as we can to deeper experiences involving all our feelings and our heart's deeper expressions, we may feel uncertain and vulnerable. It is in those moments, if we decide to remain for a time, when we also add more strength and courage into our lives.

Barbara Halcrow, MSW

Listening to Your Heart's Wisdom

> *Know that when the mind is not connected to the heart, ego rules.*
> —Kuthumi

I can say without hesitation that the heart's energy has the power to dramatically transform and soften the mind to open to thoughts of kindness, understanding, and compassion. If we leave our heart out and just listen to the mind to solve all issues, the mind tends to like to distract itself through the ego. The ego easily shifts to fear, confusion, and even disaster thinking when it's not sure about something or when it's not linked up to the heart's intuitive wisdom.

Listening to my heart has been a primary part of my inner GPS. Since early childhood, I have felt a sense of knowing from my heart, and I have tried to listen as much as possible to its intuitive voice to guide me through life's challenges.

Present-day science is now catching up with our inner spiritual knowingness, as it now recognizes that the heart actually contains a "little brain" (Braden 2015, 11–14). Specifically, the heart brain sends information electrically to our cranial brain via its own specialized neurites, which are also found in the cranial brain, in order for the heart brain to perform its many functions.

Notably, this promotes states of deeper intuition and contributes to our precognitive abilities. The heart brain can work independently from the cranial brain to provide cognition and awareness of our individual inner worlds and outer experiences. Additionally, and at minimum, the

Ultimate Self-Care

heart brain serves to provide its own independent recall and memory.

This is where the age-old phrase "wisdom of the heart" is most real and wonderful. It's what many of us have always known when looking into our hearts for guidance. In terms of intelligent collaboration, the heart also acts in harmony with the brain for tasks that benefit both organs in providing the specific service needed in each moment.

On a feeling level, how do we open our hearts more? Sometimes, we might feel we are already open enough when, in fact, we are still acting in protective ways as a habit from past rejections or pain from grief or traumatic losses. We may not be aware we have emotionally armored ourselves in an attempt to preserve some sense of safety and control. This kind of self-preservation can keep our hearts feeling unfulfilled because we are unconsciously keeping people and love at a distance.

In other moments, we open our hearts when significant losses or deaths occur. These events become triggering, painful, and transforming times where we feel cracked open to depths within ourselves, eventually to allow more healing and love to come in.

When we open our hearts more fully, all kinds of more nourishing things begin to happen. We think differently and draw in more positive events and people into our lives. We have more mind, body, and spirit energies that surge up. Our creative instincts improve, and we communicate better. We can complete projects more easily, emotional and even physical healings happen more quickly, and our immune system improves, and on it goes. The next few sections will lay out specific ways to help open your hearts.

Barbara Halcrow, MSW

Easy Heart Openings

> *What happens when people open their hearts? They get better.*
> —Haruki Murakami, *Norwegian Wood*

Think about what makes you feel happy, joyful, calm, or peaceful, or just what makes you simply smile. Think about all your senses: smell, sight, hearing, touch, taste. For example, I love the sight and smell of roses, lilacs, and carnations, especially. I love babies, animals, being by water, lying in the sun at a beach, the smell of the forest, hearing certain kinds of piano music, being with a good friend or family member, writing from my heart, watching a favorite sport, dancing, or just being outside.

As easy as this thinking sounds, as soon as you begin to think and then feel what brings you happiness, your heart, being naturally connected with your spirit and sense of love and joy, will automatically begin to open even more.

If you don' t already do this, place pictures around you of anything that uplifts you. We have pictures of our loved ones or places we love going to around us at home or at work because they are spirit lifters and heart mirrors, reminding us of the love that surrounds us and is always within us.

Quiet Focus Within

When possible, steal yourself away from overstimulation and noise to a place where you can be silent and hear your own inner voice.

- Take some deep breaths, and just look into your heart and focus on it. Our heart's true nature is full of its own gentleness, kindness, compassion, and patience. The more open our heart can be, the more we can feel a caring and accepting connection to ourselves and to all of life that surrounds us. This is where we can consciously move our mind toward more peace and calm because the loving, compassionate energy will move from the heart and infuse our mind.
- Imagine a beautiful red rose within your heart. As you focus on your heart, imagine this rose opening within your heart. Do this focus for a few seconds, and you will feel more peaceful.
- Say to yourself, "I am peace. I am love. I am compassion." Know that this affirmation for you is true.

Extending Love and Compassion

As you pass by anyone, it is easy to say within yourself, "I send you love," "I wish you well," "Much love to you," "Blessings to you," "Peace to you," or "May you be healed exactly as you need." Your silent word is still your own powerful thought command, and this brief offering of compassion and caring will go directly to that person. You might find yourself smiling soon after, with your own uplifted and lighter energy.

We can do this for people, animals, or any of earth's creatures. It also assists us in that same moment to open more to love. It can melt away any inner lingering resentment. On a more formal basis, we extend our love, compassion, and caring to others when we offer prayers on our own or in a spiritual groups or faith-based organization.

We can also choose to extend love and compassion, if only at a distance, or send a prayer to those we feel resentful toward; when we feel are able to do that, then our energy can support their strength and potential for healing.

It's more difficult to consider sending love to those we dislike or who have hurt us, but it is a radical and loving thing to do. When we send thoughts of love to those people in this way, we are sending out a higher energy, and we act to defy the lower energy vibrations of fear, resentment, and hatred.

We assume, because we cannot ever expect to see a change in someone's behavior, that when we send this energy out, nothing will ever happen.

We might not be aware of the power of a prayer or of the prayer offerings of others who are also sending their thoughts of love, light, and healing. At some point in time, our positive energy, adding to the positive energy from others, may well become the tipping point that begins to ignite a spark of conscious change and insight.

Over the years, because of the benefits of more peace of mind, I have made it a practice to work at forgiveness, of letting go anger, and to do it until I feel an honest degree of neutral energy within me. Letting go of hurt, rage, or grudges doesn't have a time frame to it; it's a very individual journey.

Gratitude

Encouraging yourself toward a sense of gratitude or thankfulness is another way of opening and expanding your heart energy. Gratitude also increases your ability to receive more abundance. Do this by simply thinking of all the things you are grateful for. When you do this, you are giving the universe permission to bring you more of the things that make you thankful.

In that instant, we are not focusing on our perceived lack of anything. For example, if you find a nickel or dime on your path, don't feel it's too small an amount to pick up; rather, retrieve it and say, "Thank you," again expressing gratitude while at the same time opening to drawing in additional universal energy to provide you with even more abundance. Expressing thankfulness raises your vibration to a higher level.

Therefore, at any point in time—or when you go to sleep and upon awakening—simply say thank you for all the things, abundance, people, and situations that support you on your life path. Think of the comfort as well as the learnings that have been brought to you.

Barbara Halcrow, MSW

Music

We know that music has a great impact on people as well as all animal and plant life. Before beginning a writing or healing session, I will put on a piece of music (piano, pan flute, harp, and guitar are my preferences) to open my heart, soften my mind, and raise my energy. In fact, during the writing of my first book as well as this one, I consistently played Doug Volz's piano in the background as I wrote.

When I need to do housework, I put on something that makes me want to move and dance. We each have our own favorites, but when it comes to what softens and calms us, we tend to be drawn to musical tones that resonate with our hearts and give our spirits a lift.

I believe our most natural balanced state is to be at peace. By opening our hearts, we begin to have an increased sense of being connected with nature or at one with the energy that surrounds us.

In this realm of acceptance, our energy expands and becomes lighter. We begin to leave the former place of stress and constriction that lowers our vibration. Moving our vibration upwards expands the real strength and power in the attributes of love: compassion, kindness, empathy, and forgiveness.

David Hawkins in *Power vs. Force* (2012) says it well: "Power is what makes you strong, while force makes you go weak. Love, compassion and forgiveness, which may be mistakenly seen by some as submissive, are in fact profoundly empowering" (162).

Forgiveness

What does forgiveness mean? It means to consciously choose to let go and lose interest in continuously reliving a history where anger and hatred reside. "It is letting go of the desire to hurt others or ourselves because of something that is already in the past" (Jampolsky 2007, 17).

Letting go of resentments of any nature can be hard work if they've been there awhile. To forgive is to free ourselves emotionally and spiritually because it allows us to live more fully in the present moment, with far more calmness. For me, forgiveness or the letting go of anger, resentment, or grudges is necessary to keep my heart unblocked and open. Forgiveness, in some instances, takes years to resolve, depending on different factors.

I can say that depending on the impact of the emotional injury, forgiveness is generally not a one-time practice. It can be a frequent and necessary process if we find remnants of grudges that continue to be triggered. Those triggers will tell us that we are not finished releasing resentment, hurt, or a loss of some kind.

No matter how small the inner active hurt or grudge, it can still lower our energy because it can create an energy block, a sore, and it will keep returning to us to be healed. Sores have a way of festering when left unattended and can develop into more serious issues or even manifest as physical ailments.

There are also moments when we realize that even more than forgiving someone else, we need to stop being so angry at ourselves and forgive ourselves for being caught in a situation that felt injurious to us, or where we felt we consciously made the wrong decision and got hurt by the result.

What I've found helpful in my own healing processes is to come to a place where I can see the strengths and goodness in others, no matter what I feel has happened, and to look with compassion in that they, too, have their own journey full of hazards, mistakes, and painful lessons. They, too, have the same universal source of energy within them, and on that level, we all are connected, even if we don't wish to be. As part of my Reiki training, we do acknowledge the divinity within all of us, and this understanding connects us all throughout our human family. Remembering this acknowledgment when I am struggling to find compassion when my ego has felt offended has been extremely beneficial to me, helping me to regain my sense of connectedness to everyone on this planet.

Some people will wake up after a life-altering event and discover a kinder, more compassionate part of themselves has emerged. They then decide to pass on their learning. Others have a different journey to follow but can also be teachers for us. Their difficult and sometimes injurious behavior can move us to stand our ground with far more strength and backbone, playing a catalytic role in promoting our personal growth.

Remembering Our Innocence

Another thing we can do to help move us toward acceptance, forgiveness, and more peace is to remind ourselves of the innocent person we all are inside, regardless of what has happened in our lives that may block us from achieving a

Ultimate Self-Care

fuller connection to our Creator, or the source of universal love. I feel that adopting this perception benefits us once again in allowing our hearts to be more open, which I believe is really our more natural state of being.

Sometimes, when we know of someone who has a really distasteful personality or, in a more extreme example, has committed some heinous act, like Hitler, Jeffery Dahmer, or Clifford Olson, we will search for some reason for it and ask, "What happened to them? Who or what kind of beliefs brought them to do what they did? What were they like as a child and how were they treated? Was a there a void of love for them?" We recognize that something came into play that took them away from a more natural, loving state of innocence and a sense of ethics and morality.

If you are able to go back in time to your childhood photos and follow your life path in pictures up through the ages, you will see your core innocence and the fact you were most likely always curious to learn more about yourself, or to at least be given the chance to find what path felt right for you. You may well see that you still have the pureness of heart that loves the simple, joyful things in life. You can also experience that same sense of innocence that can be reflected back to you in the unconditional love and innocence from animals, babies, and children.

If we are at odds with someone, we can also think of him or her in a state of innocence as a child. While that thought might never make you want to spend any further time with the individual, it can help dissolve some degree of resentment.

Barbara Halcrow, MSW

Forgiveness Exercise

Based on my own experiences, I believe that holding grudges does not allow me to have the degree of openheartedness I need to bring me the peace I seek. Forgiveness has become a necessity. Forgiveness does not always mean we will simply forget what happened, but it can mean that the incident or situation we experienced as painful will not have the same negative power to hold us back or influence how we move our lives forward. The following mindfulness exercise should never be felt as a strain; it is meant as a suggestion, a gentle guide, whereby you may create one that may fit you better. It can be done as many times as you wish, and you can create your own exercises over time.

Breathe in and out slowly, and ground yourself in the moment. Visualize a bubble of white light completely surrounding you, like an egg shape. This is your energy shield; no negative energy is able to penetrate it.

Only when you are ready, think of the person you feel has hurt you. See them sitting or standing before you. You may or may not fully understand the reason for the person's actions toward you, but you can say this:

I don't like what you did, and I accept what has happened. I now choose to move forward in my life.

I accept you as you are, and I forgive you for your actions.

I accept and forgive the situation; I let go of what happened.

I move on to greater strength.

I move on to greater wisdom.

I move on to greater love.

Ultimate Self-Care

May you find the healing you need with our Creator.
May you find peace within yourself.
May you find the love that resides within you.
May you be able to bring more love into this world.

Being released from resentment helps us to connect back to our hearts and have a greater sense of inner peace.

Staying Present in the Moment

Eckhart Tolle has written significantly on being present. Try this experiment offered in Tolle's 1999 book, *The Power of Now:*

> Close your eyes and say to yourself: "I wonder what my next thought is going to be?"
>
> Then become very alert and wait for your next thought. Be like a cat watching a mouse hole. What thought is going to come out of the mouse hole? Try it now. "Well?" (93)

Those who tried this exercise will likely comment that it took a while for a thought to arrive. Tolle remarks, "As long as you are in a state of intense presence you are free of thought. You are still, yet highly alert. The instant your conscious attention sinks below a certain level, thought rushes in. The mental noise returns. The stillness is lost. You are back in time" (94).

Being present does not feel like an easy thing to do most of the time, nor do we think of practicing this state of consciousness very often. Often, we find ourselves moving

Barbara Halcrow, MSW

from one thought or one activity to another. We try to stay on top things as we attempt to slow down the momentum of any fears or challenges that are vying for our attention.

Tolle and others who extensively practice the art of meditation speak of the need to be grounded in our bodies to initiate a greater state of being present. The focus on deep breathing into our bodies is a key to being more present, calm, and relaxed (see chapter 3).

Managing Fear and Anxiety in the Moment

We cannot maintain an open heart, hear our own spiritual guidance, or feel the compassion for others when we are immersed in fear and anxiety. Degrees of fear and feelings of love cannot coexist in one moment. The fastest way I know of calming myself in a moment of stress, fear, or anxiety is to breathe deeply. Taking several deep breaths to calm your mind and body works immediately. If need be, with each inhalation, you can add these statements, which I have learned throughout my spiritual studies and found effective over time:

"I breathe in strength. I breathe out fear. I breathe in courage. I breathe out fear. I breathe in calm. I breathe out fear. I breathe in love. I breathe out fear.

"I am loved."

You can also tell yourself:

"I am kindness. I am empathy. I am compassion. I am strength. I am eternal."

When you say these statements, you are connecting with your spiritual nature, and you are aligning with what is spiritually known as the "I Am presence" within, or what's also referred to as your Higher Self. If we can return for a time to affirm those strong qualities, we have within us, we can help to rebalance and calm ourselves.

Cocreating What We Already Deserve

We are cocreating our lives with the universal energies around us; we use our energy in our thoughts, words, beliefs, and actions to manifest what we want to see unfold in our lives. Cocreation becomes a greater reality when we consider we are in an energy exchange with the same powerful, intelligent, loving energy that surrounds us and runs throughout our world.

We begin our journeys in different degrees of privilege and circumstance, and we have our own evolving paths of challenges and spiritual learning. If we feel we are not quite on our right path, where we don't feel a sense of passion about where we are at, it doesn't mean something is wrong; it means we are still learning to feel our way through. Remembering to be a kind, loving, and compassionate human being will always be an extremely powerful way to live your life. It is, in itself, a path of the heart that makes a difference to everyone you connect with.

This world can be unquestionably challenging at times. It does not serve us to judge ourselves in any way or to compare ourselves to others who appear to be far more successful. It helps us to be reflective in acknowledging our courage, strength, and resilience in the difficulties we have already overcome and to go forward from there.

What we can also do is take what we know about ourselves and see if we can make changes that feel doable.

If we check into our daily self-talk and listen closely, we will hear where we are affirming ourselves, positively or negatively. All of those thoughts and feelings impact our self-esteem and energy levels and determine how we move ourselves toward what we want to see happen in our lives.

We might start out by thinking of having a better job or relationship, but then we might catch ourselves thinking that maybe we aren't quite good enough to receive it or don't really deserve it or some other self-doubt. In that case, we might not take any action to shift us in the direction we really want to go.

If we want a chance to see changes in some of our circumstances, we can start with working to shift any false beliefs or thought patterns about our sense of worthiness. We also need to be discerning about who we spend our time with. Some people do not really have our best interests at heart and are not genuinely interested in our success or our well-being; their energy, influence, and messages can be eroding. We have all met these people. The ones who don't keep your confidence, who are overtly competitive with you, who don't or can't make time to listen to you. Good relationships are not perfect; they have moments of discord and learning, but they are about seeking balance, appreciation, and an honest reciprocity.

The best action we can take is to maintain, as often as possible, a deeper, steadfast appreciation of who we are in our gifts, skills, and strengths and by continuing to express who we are, without unrealistic notions of needing to be perfect. I feel that to truly believe that we all deserve to receive the best that life has to offer is a powerful singular thought.

If there are any areas of inner turmoil or resentment, then this is where our focus needs to be to develop more inner peace. Cocreation doesn't just involve thinking and feeling what we want; it also involves using the information that's just been written regarding opening your heart, extending gratitude and compassion, working on acceptance, and letting go of judgments we hold about ourselves and about others we feel have harmed us. This certainly has been, and continues to be, my own greatest challenge.

If our inner life can be more peaceful, it can also make the energy we put forward on our own behalf much stronger and more magnetizing. When we let go of inner emotional baggage, we feel more energized and begin to move more quickly in the direction we want to go. We begin to see that we can create better circumstances for ourselves when we can feel and know, more decisively, we truly deserve to have them.

There are other benefits. When we clear away more inner blocks like resentment, guilt, shame, blame, and other things that lower our energy, we find more of our senses come alive. We become more sensitively tuned in to ourselves and to all of nature. We hear and see things more deeply. Our intuitive gifts become acute, and we experience our life with more joy and lightness of heart.

Overall, it becomes essential that we seek to love and care for ourselves as much as we can.

Barbara Halcrow, MSW

Three Guiding Questions

1. "How May I Best Serve?"

I have found the simple question, "How may I best serve?" to be particularly useful when looking at changes I want to manifest in my own career path. It is a question posed to one's loving higher self (the part of you most directly connected to the divine or universal intelligence). It is a way to be guided toward my highest good in giving service to humanity, a service that allows me to fulfill my gifts and creative energies in a way that brings me greater happiness and meets my financial needs.

When we ask this question, it allows us to be guided to the best path without needlessly worrying about our ego's concern about how our choices may appear to others. We are perfectly open to receive the information that comes to us.

I learned to ask this question at various times in my life as I grew and changed my occupational pursuits. It was provided to me from a spiritually reflective book called *Teachings of Silver Birch*: "The power that is behind you is the power of the Great Spirit in all of life, the greatest force in the universe. That power must manifest and you can help it to bring its force into your world. It does not matter what you do—whether you raise one up, whether you give a word of encouragement, whether you serve in things of spirit or things of matter—as long as you serve and you are not weary of service, you are instruments of the Great Spirit" (Silver Birch 2002, 196).

The information reflects that when we are pursuing our soul's highest calling, in whatever vocation or service,

Ultimate Self-Care

whether it be simple or complex in nature, all of the service we give is important when we give and interact from the heart.

2. "What Would a Wise Person Do?"

This is another simple question to help you to quickly draw up your own deeper wisdom when facing challenging situations and you need clarity for the right path or action to take. In a moment of quiet, just ask, and you may find the answer comes quickly.

3. Will My Action Show Respect for Myself?

Asking this question brings an immediate answer. If we say, "No, it doesn't show respect for myself," and we carry on with the action anyway, we may have an addiction or overattachment to something, a situation, person, or substance, or maybe our boundaries are weak. A simple example is when you know you need to rest, as you've been overextended at work, but your friend calls and wants to go out for dinner and chat. You love dining out, even though it can be pricy, and don't want to disappoint your friend, so you agree to go out instead of laying low for the evening and getting the sleep your system needs.

We are sometimes anxious to make a decision on behalf of our own self-care; we are afraid to say no, for whatever reason. It is good to ask, "Will my action show respect for myself?" If we don't get a clear, immediate answer it's good to step back and sit with the question for a few minutes before making a decision, or talk to someone to get some clarity.

Barbara Halcrow, MSW

A Manifesting Process

If we believe, feel, visualize, and affirm something we want often enough, it will most likely manifest in some form. If this does not come easy for you, here are some helpful guidelines for positive cocreation:

- Be very clear about what you want, because you are giving the universal energy a specific command. The universe responds precisely and fastest when your mind is clear and decisive.
- List the specific details describing what you want, because as you study it once a day, you will impress your wishes on your deeper unconscious mind.
- Feel what it is you want and how it feels to receive it.
- Get a good mental visualization of what you want.
- Find a physical representation of what you want via a picture or drawing or smaller replica that will add to the strength of your project.
- Ensure that what you are seeking is aligned with your highest good and does not harm you or anyone or anything else. Let it be based on knowing you truly deserve the best that life has to offer.
- Keep as silent as possible about what you are doing in your creation so the energy can quietly build up inside you, creating a stronger magnetic pull from the energies that surround you.
- Be ready and open to receive what you want, and visualize it happening.

Ultimate Self-Care

- Become present in your imagination and affirm you have now received what you want (e.g., "I now have a new job opportunity, and I feel great").
- Let it go. Let your request go and continue on with your day. Take it easy, knowing that all things come in the right time and the right way, when we are ready to receive them. Some things can take years to arrive, but when they do, the timing makes sense to us in retrospect.
- Act on any intuitive ideas, nudges, or messages that you receive. When you take a step forward, the universe will automatically illuminate the next step for you.
- Try to remain patient as things unfold; it's only the ego part of us that gets scared and overly demanding. Just tell it that everything's going in the right way. Go outside, play, relax, and then continue to listen to your intuitive self for the next step.
- Love and care for yourself as much as you can.

Know that the universal energy that we are connected into is loving and supportive in nature and constantly works with us to help us achieve the successful outcome we deserve. This is one of the most important things to keep in mind. I have had moments of doubt, as anyone does, when venturing into unfamiliar territory.

As you have read in this book, I also experienced successful outcomes by choosing to remind myself to trust in the nature of this loving, intelligent energy that lies within us and all around us, because it will continually attempt to provide for us in the ways we need to be successful. It will nudge us and give us subtle signals as to our next moves. We just need to take time to relax our minds, listen, and follow in taking any small steps that come to mind toward our goal. The more we trust ourselves, our natural gifts, our imagination, our visual abilities, and the power of our own thoughts and words, the faster we will manifest, and the less it becomes a formula to follow. [17]

Affirmations for Health and Wellness

> *Affirmations are our mental vitamins, providing the supplementary positive thoughts we need to balance the barrage of negative events and thoughts we experience daily.*
> —Tia Walker (with Peggi Speers)

I believe that positive affirmations are our own power statements and act like specific commandments to the universal energies.

In essence, as spiritual beings, they are our inherited right to proclaim, to use our words in the correct way, to bring about positive changes. The following are some examples of daily affirmations that can strengthen you:

- Every day in every way, I am getting healthier and stronger.
- I am confident in my ability to manage all situations that come my way.

---

[17] There are countless CDs, books, and downloads from the internet that offer guidance for cocreating, manifesting, and developing your own personal affirmations. For further resources, see appendix C.

Ultimate Self-Care

- I develop habits that support a healthy lifestyle.
- I am creative, intelligent, strong, and youthful.
- I respect myself.
- I am open to receiving all the abundance life has to offer.
- I deserve to receive everything I need, and that brings me happiness.
- There is enough abundance for us all.

Synchronicity

Synchronicity is an ever-present reality for those who have eyes to see.

—Carl Jung

Synchronicity is part of our cocreation and manifestation processes. As you proceed on your day, you'll notice the coincidences that come into your life to guide you in the way you want to go. These include those so-called chance encounters with people who give you guidance or information just when you need it, or when you get flashes of insight to contact someone who helps you.

I returned to Vancouver after teaching English in Seoul, Korea, for fourteen months and had to find a place to live. I was temporarily staying with a friend, but he had little space, and I wanted to get re-established. As I searched, I saw the vacancy rate in Vancouver at the time was next to nil. I felt somewhat lost and couldn't figure out my next move, so I just lay down to rest. Suddenly, a woman's name popped into my head, someone I'd not spoken to for a long time. I knew I had to call her. She immediately told me someone next door to her was moving out, and she was also friends with the landlord and would arrange an interview. Luckily, the suite hadn't been advertised, as the rent was very reasonable, and my friend also knew someone who could paint it at a low cost to brighten it up. I got the suite, and the location couldn't have been better, right near the ocean in Vancouver.

Synchronicities can also be when you see words on a sign, books that come into your possession, images you see, or songs you happen to hear at the right time to give you clues for actions you can take or validation that you are simply on the right path.

This is the supportive, loving universe communicating with you in ways to get your attention, letting you know you are heard and it's there to support and assist you. This is what being in the flow is about. It is essentially allowing yourself to put your effort forward in terms of using your imagination, visualization, and affirmations clearly, and then letting it all go, and not pushing or forcing anything, just allowing yourself to gently feel the energies around you that are helping you.

This is the area of trusting that things will work out if you stay with it. This process can test our patience, but we also need to allow the timing involved to unfold, in receiving what we need or want.

Sometimes, there are other signals we may begin to see, like repeating numbers. Repeating numbers in threes and fours, such as 111, 222, 333, 444, and 555, have appeared around me on a daily basis for years to signal, for example, that I am on the right path. When I see them, I notice what I have just been thinking. It can be a clue to a meaning.

Ultimate Self-Care

There are no coincidences here, as numbers represent universal vibrations in their energy patterns, and it's up to us to figure out how to read the energy signals. If you talk to people about number sequences, you might find to your surprise that you have company for discussion.

Many people, including my close friends and others along my journey, have mentioned they are noticing an increase in this phenomenon; some attribute it to the increased connection to our higher selves. It can also mean we are receiving the guidance of the angelic realm more directly, indicating there is more assistance being given at this time on earth.[18]

I have always looked for signals during my life, with all forms of nature. I have often lived near parks or spent time out in nature. I have received specific kinds of warnings and greetings of joy from songbirds and other birds, such as crows, eagles, robins, and owls. One time, a crow visited me on the corner of my balcony, which was unusual because my apartment was on a high level, and I mostly received visits from seagulls.

The crow suddenly cawed so loudly that its sound reverberated throughout my apartment, leaving me feeling stunned. I believe crows can portend types of deaths or transitions. As it happened, my beloved cat was ailing and had a grand mal seizure only a day afterwards, which was

---

[18] Doreen Virtue, *Angel Numbers 101: The Meaning of 111, 123, 444, and Other Number Sequences* (Hay House, 2008); Joanne, "Sacred Scribes, Repetitive Numbers Sequences, Angel Numbers." http://sacredscribesangelnumbers.blogspot.com/p/index-numbers.html; Ramona Remestat, "Angel Numbers Decoder Guide." https://ramonaremesat.com/wp-content/uploads/2017/12/Angel-Number-De-Coder-BONUS.pdf

Barbara Halcrow, MSW

a signal of her need to pass on to spirit. I feel this crow's appearance was letting me know in advance of my cat's severe condition and need to pass on. I knew it was a matter of time she had to leave, and I was having difficulty letting her go.

Other land or sea animals or even insects who suddenly appear, seemingly out of place or when least expected, can hold meaning and provide thoughtful pause as a signal for me. After my initial life's fear of spiders, I have learned over time that they are powerful symbols, warning me to not get entangled in certain situations or relationships. These appearances have been invaluable to me in also connecting to how I am really feeling about a situation. It is good to reflect inside what animals, birds, or insects hold meaning for you, those nature beings that you feel emotionally or spiritually close to, or even repelled by. Their attributes can be helpful in any of the messages they are bringing forward.

Overall, the universe knows what kind of signals make sense to each of us in following our paths, and the more we choose to notice, the more often we will see them.

CHAPTER 8

SELF-CARE BECOMES GLOBAL CARE

Every conscious act toward supporting our own self-care continues on as an active positive energy that ripples outward, adding nourishing vitality throughout our homes and into our communities. The more we extend and build on the energy of love through kindness and compassion, the more it grows and has a positive influence on our environment.

When we go forward in loving self-care, we become increasingly conscious of the ways we can responsibly harvest, replenish, and sustain our earth. We become invested in knowing the earth is also being given utmost regard in land and soil conservation practices to yield the highest quality of food.

We care more about the quantity, quality, and conservation reserves of our water. We are concerned about the air we breathe. If we consume animals or use animal by-products, we find out about the animal's well-being in their quality of life and their end of life. Many more people are now transitioning away from animal consumption as we become conscious of the needless suffering and cruelty towards animals and the destructive impact of the meat packing industry on our planet's health.

When we pay attention to the ways we show love and respect for ourselves, we also notice all manner of industries, services, and legislative bodies that provide for us. We want to know that they are accountable in upholding the sanctity of life by developing policies, practices, and procedures that contribute to our and the planet's well-being.

Moreover, as we continue to move and open our hearts and minds in this positive direction, many of us will experience our lives shifting in other ways. We will understand people with deeper and clearer perceptions, and we will feel the cord of our universal connectedness.

We will also feel an even greater depth of caring for all life on earth. Some will feel this connection to animals more profoundly as we embrace the fact that we are all sentient beings in our own unique physical, emotional, and spiritual senses. We will be able to look into the eyes of an animal and feel its soul. We will consider the creatures of the sea, like whales and dolphins, and when we enter the waters of their home, we will realize these soulful, cultural, and intelligent beings may instinctively have an awareness of who we are more than we realize.

We will view insects and reptiles that we once found uninteresting or even frightening and easily sense their innate intelligence. Our ability to more fully connect with creatures, plants, and all of earth's life forms will become an ongoing source of respectful curiosity, learning, and joy. We will begin to sense the remarkable intelligence and synchronistic beauty of our earth.

The Earth Is an Intelligent Being

When we spend time in nature, we can feel that special energy all around us, energy we love and find spiritually rejuvenating. We can regain more of our own inner peace when we take in the healing energy the earth gives.

Many of us reflect on this energy when we're at our desk and think about being by the ocean or hiking, some place that takes us to our natural grounded sense of connection. When we spend time with earth, we are with a mother source. That experience is true, in a way, because we contain the very elements of earth. Our energy is connected to the earth through our hearts and spiritual centers as well.

From an energetic and spiritual perspective, researchers like Robert Coon, who authored *Earth Chakras: The Definitive Guide* (2009), also recognize that our earth is a living being that has its own life chakra energy system, just as we do. Coon states, "The Earth is alive, with its own chakra and circulatory system. Great ley arteries transmit vitalizing forces around the world through major sacred sites, advancing the evolution of all life" (http://earthchakras.org/Introduction.php).

Coon cites the seven main earth chakra locations on the planet:[19]

First Chakra (Root): Mount Shasta, California

This chakra is considered to be primal in generating earth's life force, prior to life assuming biological form.

---

[19] Robert Coon, http://earthchakras.org/Locations.php

Second Chakra: Lake Titicaca, Peru and Bolivia

This high elevation center's dual purpose has been to regulate new species on the earth as well as the major evolutionary advancements for life.

Third Chakra: Uluru-Kata Tjuta, Northern Territory, Australia

This enormous monolithic rock, also known as Ayers Rock, acts like the earth's solar plexus. This rock acts to maintain, energize, and increase the health of all in the area.

Fourth Chakra: Glastonbury and Shaftesbury, England

These locations in England act like earth's heart chakra and are thought to be the home of the Holy Grail. This high, spiritual vortex is purposeful in opening our hearts and raising the frequency of all life forms, as well as encouraging individuals globally toward more love and compassion.

Fifth Chakra: Great Pyramid, Mt. Sinai, Mt. of Olives, and Middle East

This is considered to be the throat or voice of earth's spirit, centrally located in the whole of our landmass. Its purpose is to align us with earth's spirit, to connect with her directly in order to understand her will for all dependent upon her.

Sixth Chakra: Aeon Activation Chakra

Like our pineal gland in the human brain that activates us to perceive energy and life more deeply, this chakra is an activation center that helps humankind to perceive the other dimensions of our earth and show how we can participate in advancement of life in its many forms over longer periods.

Seventh Chakra: Mount Kailas, Tibet

The Crown Chakra, Mt. Kailas, is the roof of the world. Considering the high spiritual teachings the Tibetan people have brought to humankind, one can see a powerful energy that is meant to be instrumental in allowing the individual purpose and earth's evolutionary purpose to be unified. This unification is dedicated to overcoming the decline of life and spiritual death, to the understanding of our eternal spiritual nature.

If we look at each of the chakra sites as laid out by Coon, and if we have had opportunity to travel to any of these main energy power centers, we will most likely feel that any of these centers have prompted deeper insights and changes for us. Many times, we are drawn to various places on this planet for that very reason; we are resonating an energy that begins to pull us to the very place we need to go to make that deeper connection with ourselves.

There are other key points on our planet that when we visit, we tell ourselves, "I know this place," "I feel I've been here before," or "I feel at home." I lived in the Yukon Territory and spent time in Egypt, the United Kingdom, and Sedona, Arizona; I felt a strong spiritual connection to these locations. There are other places in the world that I long to travel to because I instinctively know they are areas that will enrich my soul.

Robert Coon and other authors tell us there is so much more to our planet as an entire complex energy body than the knowledge of the earth's chakras. There is far more information about the kinds of intelligent, interconnecting energy systems of our earth than the reader can explore.

The Earth's Intelligence in Sacred Designs

One cannot help but take pause at the brilliance and beauty of specific designs found throughout our natural universe. I am referring to the geometric designs that not only reflect how our form as human beings is constructed but are also part of the geometric matrix of the entire universe.

The following drawing of the ancient figure of the Flower of Life has been studied over thousands of years and is recognized mathematically as containing all the elements involved in creation of matter, time, and space.

In his writings contained in *The Ancient Secret of the Flower of Life, Volume 1* (1998), Drunvalo Melchizedek relays the clarity he received regarding the energetic geometric meaning of the Flower of Life while at the ancient site at Abydos by stating, "This design contains in its proportions, every single aspect of life there is. It contains every mathematical formula, law of physics, every harmony in music, and every biological life-form right down to your specific body. It contains every atom, every dimensional level, absolutely everything that's within wave form universes" (29).

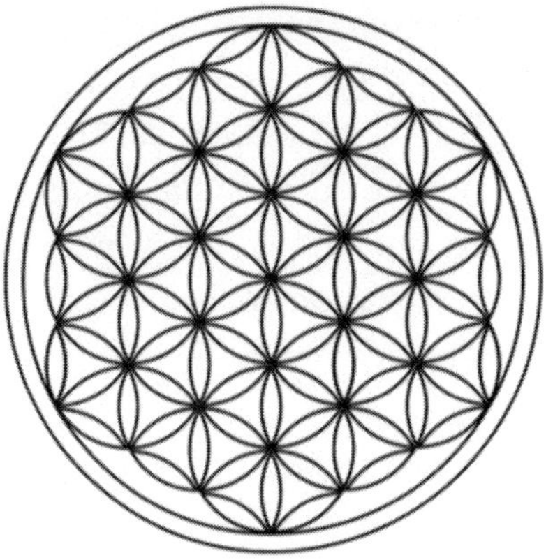

Ultimate Self-Care

Figure 1. Flower of Life
(Alexandra Barbu, https://www.dreamstime.com)

Several years ago, I had the opportunity to travel to Egypt on a sacred spiritual journey; we visited many powerful spiritual centers of Egypt's ancient origins.

In visiting Abydos, I came upon the same drawing of the Flower of Life as Melchizedek. The Egyptologist informed us that this drawing in this particular location is thought to be one of the oldest on the planet. The design of the Flower of Life was burned into the stone at Abydos; it was barely visible from the distance where I stood while photographing it. Unfortunately, it cannot be visually reproduced clearly enough to include in this book.

Many of us will automatically recognize this design as a symbol found in many worldwide religions as well as in our mathematical symbols. Mathematics is a universal language, and the Flower of Life symbol is a part of sacred mathematical geometry. Geometry and mathematical ratios, harmonics, and proportions are also found in music, light, and cosmology (Melchizedek 1998, 41).

Most of us studied geometry in our earlier school years, learning mathematical principles and applications when we looked at triangles, cubes, and circles. I'm sure we had no idea we were working with earth's most sacred blueprints.

Melchizedek essentially purports throughout his writing that sacred geometry opens doors to higher consciousness when one begins to closely examine these ancient designs. This perspective actually began long ago with the Greeks, who placed foundational value in their belief that "geometry and numbers are sacred because they codify the hidden order behind creation. They are the instruments used to create the physical universe" (Skinner 2006, 15).

In nature, geometric designs are abundant. Spirals are only one example, and they can be easily found in the horns of animals or in shells like the chambered nautilus in Figure 2. On a massive scale, we can view them in the giant galaxy in Figure 3, an example of our own spiral Milky Way galaxy. Both figures appear to show the same geometric logarithm at play, which is also a fractal (Ibid., 58).

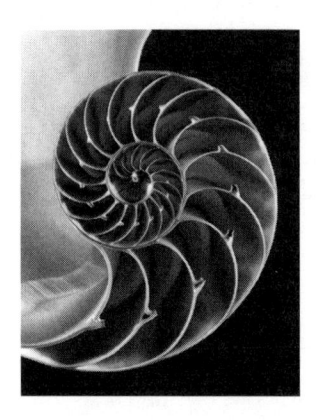

Figure 2: Nautilus Shell Interior
(Christian Delbert, https://www.dreamstime.com)

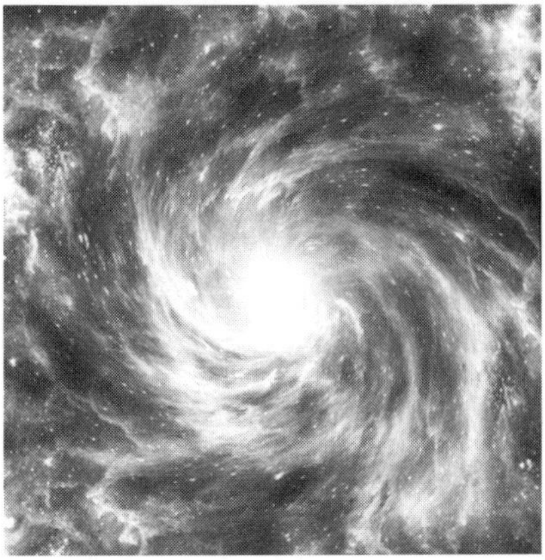

Figure 3: Spiral Galaxy
(Grytisaj, https://www.dreamstime.com

These natural and consistently repeating recursive designs are also referred to as fractals. You can see many of them easily, as they are all around us in tree leaves, pine cones, broccoli, ferns, and even shorelines when viewed from high above.

Some of the geometric replications also come through great works of art. In past centuries, an understanding of the geometry of perspective was necessary for the production of great art and great architecture (Skinner 2006, 89). That perspective is still true today of many art and architectural forms.

Many artists throughout time have been spiritually drawn to replicate nature through their meditations. Such is the case of those artists producing relatively precise geometric art forms – many primarily by freehand. In the creation of these designs as well as in viewing them, it allows any of us to access deeper parts of our consciousness and it can provide healing. Examples of sacred geometry are found in the inspirational sacred geometric mandala designs from two artists below.

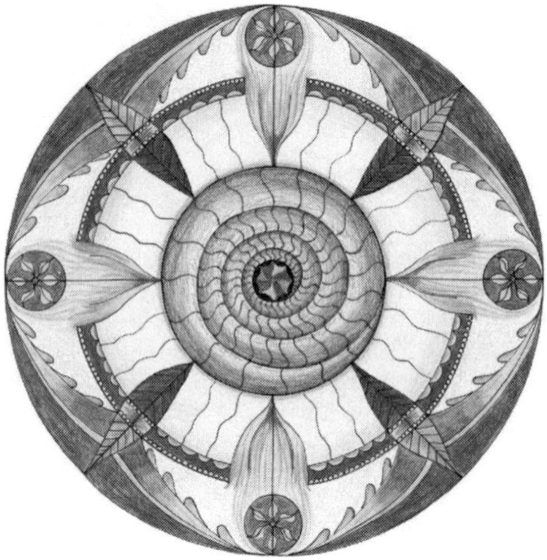

Figure 4. Sacred Geometric Mandala

Meg MacQueen, a holistic health coach (www.Megmacqueen.com), said, "These mandalas are hand-drawn intuitively, and radiate a vortex of harmonizing energy; each one is 'alive.' Each is unique and created with pure intention and infused with energy. The design is natural and universal and connects with us on a cellular level. They radiate energy even when simply hanging on a wall and can support healing when used as a meditation tool. The act of drawing a mandala can also be a healing experience and a powerful tool of expression."

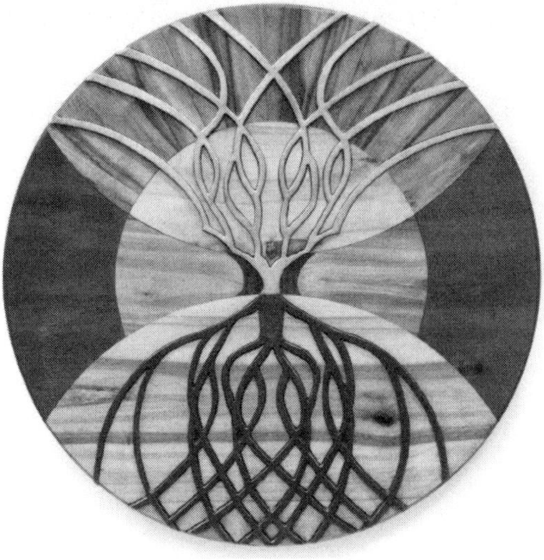

Ultimate Self-Care

Figure 5. The Tree of Cosmic Self-Knowledge
(www.clairemurgatroyd.com)

In Figure 5, with regard to her art designs, Murgatroyd states, "I use my art practice to develop and evolve a personal magical system. "The Tree of Cosmic Self-Knowledge' includes the symbolism of intertwining tree branches above and below the earth's horizon. The branches represent different time-lines of past life experiences. The semi-precious stone amber, fossilized resin from the sap of ancient trees, represents our inner spark and ancient connection to the universal source" (www.clairemurgatroyd.com).

We can see the prevailing universal intelligence in these few but compelling examples of telluric designs through the creative connection and love expressed by artists. When we embrace the earth in a heart-sense way, our artistry flows through in beautiful synchronicity.

Earth's expressions of her creations are precise, intricate, delicate, and powerful in their scope, beyond time and space. As we notice these shapes throughout our earth and recognize the being, we are living upon, we naturally want to ensure there is no harm created to our planet or its inhabitants.

What Earth Needs

In 1992, NASA astronaut Jack Lousma was on the Skylab Space Station; as the president and chief executive officer of the Centre for International Earth Science Information Network, in experiencing the powerful view of Earth from space, he wrote the following as part of his Preface in *Pathways of Understanding: The Interactions of Humanity and Global Environmental Change*:

> This experience also makes us realize that Earth itself is a kind of spacecraft, and we are all astronauts upon it, hurtling along at amazing speed. Just as the inhabitants of a spacecraft must conserve supplies, keep their ship clean and strive to work together in harmony, we must do the same on Spacecraft Earth. If we are to enjoy a safe and successful mission, we must use our resources wisely, be good stewards of our environment and strive to improve our relationships. (2, par. 3)

Earth needs what we need: loving energy, respect, care, protection, and support to flourish and evolve. The earth

Ultimate Self-Care

responds in various ways to our human activities, as she does to all other life forms. We are in an ever-evolving, synergistic, and profoundly sacred relationship with our planet.

As a living, sentient being that is made up of countless interrelated diverse ecological systems, the earth has a kind of conscious awareness of our collective energies where we gather in our communities. As our conscious awareness is increasing, we are also uplifting many parts of our world's ecological systems, replenishing them with improved, environmentally sound practices.

Unfortunately, there is still a high degree of imbalance of our planet's environment that can render negative results for all of life, unless we cooperatively forge a clear and persistent path for earth's recovery. Although restorative efforts are being made, more needs to happen. [20]

In December 2015, world leaders became galvanized around global warming issues, and from that endeavor, the Paris Agreement on climate action was adopted, with the main action plan focused on the steps needed to limit global warming to well below 2 degrees Celsius and achieve zero-net emission by the second half of the twenty-first century

(Paris Agreement/Climate Action,
http://ec.europa.eu/clima/policies/international/negotiations).

---

[20] A website to a brief video on earth's possible future changes (December 11, 2013, Mischa Reuben): *The Earth's Next 100 Years, Visualized*, Upworthy (https://www.upworthy.com/the-future-of-the-earth-s-next-100-years-visualized).

Barbara Halcrow, MSW

With differing and changing political perceptions of what this global change initiative can mean economically or otherwise, some countries may not wish to carry through in their full commitment to this global agreement. However, this legally binding agreement was the first of its kind in human history and will need to be decisively carried forward.

We know that although the challenges our global community is facing are serious, each one of us can make a difference in contributing to our earth's replenishment. There appears to be far greater public and political will being harnessed to push us forward in the necessary steps.

Listening to the Indigenous Peoples

Although the reference below was written many years ago, the knowledge and prophecies of Indigenous peoples are still relevant today.

> The reason the Earth changes are happening, and will continue to happen, is because many humans are not yet willing to make necessary changes in themselves and their actions, which could prevent them. They are not willing to stop polluting and to start moving in a sacred manner. They will not stop throwing their garbage all over the planet. (Sun Bear, Wabun Wind, 1992, 51)

Indigenous peoples over time have watched and warned us of what we need to consider with these forthcoming changes. As original caretakers of the earth, Indigenous peoples have long held the sacred and holistic belief that there is an intimate connection between the health of the earth and the health of the person.

This means in all bio-diverse ways, the earth must be honored and protected from air, water, and soil pollutants. The earth needs to be preserved in a manner that respects healthy resource development and uses conservation practices that preserve the integrity of all life forms. Earth does not exist simply for the taking. Whatever is needed, only that amount should be removed or extracted in a way that does not harm the earth's elements or her ability to be replenished, all to ensure future generations can also be fully nourished. Preserving the earth's health will help us and all living entities live in balance and avoid further depletions or mass extinctions.

Unfortunately, we know that around the world, Indigenous people's holistic beliefs and practices have not been followed in the advent of the global industrialization processes affecting trade, culture, environment, and technology. As all peoples and life forms on the planet are now being exposed to untold numbers of contaminants and pollutants, it becomes vital that we listen to the Indigenous people's understanding and their ability to provide a necessary perspective in the need for cooperative stewardship. In developing respectful policies and sound methods of eco-systemic resource and conservation management and humanity's overall conscious awakening, we will, step by step, gain ground in upholding earth's and humanity's recovery. We will have far fewer missteps when we become more conscious of the impact on our earth with every decision we make.

Barbara Halcrow, MSW

How Individual Self-Care Affects Earth's Health

It's important to take time to know our own planet, to take an active interest in connecting with it by spending time in observing and finding out how you really feel in different settings. Digging your feet into the soil, being out on the waterways, watching and listening to the earth's creatures and plants, and looking up at the sky and stars, are simple ways that bring us closer to earth's energies in those very moments. Experiencing what this planet really gives us is truly profound. This planet is essentially a planet of love because nature is filled with loving creations and energies. We have forgotten who we are in our true energetic connectedness with this magnificent being. Moving away from our sense of separateness, of insensitive detachment from our planet, as being a thing rather than a living being, will bring us closer to a sense of being connected to the earth. I believe this perspective of the interconnection with our planet is as crucial to the future and the evolutionary well-being of the earth as it is to our own.

The ways we nourish our minds, emotions, bodies, and spirits has an impact on our planet. What we give to our earth will be given back to us. We have a natural reciprocity that is part of the dynamic relationship between humanity and earth. When we nourish the earth well, as we would nourish a dear friend, the earth will respond with increased energy in what she produces. If we consider this kind of reciprocal relationship, then we can come into an increased sense of our interconnectedness, a sense of oneness with our planet's living energy.

Ultimate Self-Care

Therefore, the ways and means we produce our food, what foods we choose to eat, and how we store our food and dispose of our waste have a constant impact on our planet. Further, our personal behaviors in how we cope with our feelings and stress levels, and how we spend time entertaining ourselves, as well as what we purchase to wear and how we rid ourselves of unwanted belongings, are also factors. These areas and more have a direct impact on our health and our planet's health. Considering most of us want to do what's best for ourselves and for the earth, we can make informed, conscious choices to support our own and our planet's health in some key areas. Here are a few tips:

Mental health: We know that spending time in nature is good for our mental health. However, our mental health can also have an impact on earth's health. What we view, the people we choose to connect with, and the kinds of stimulation that negatively affects us can influence how we feel and behave. Ways to maintain good mental health in keeping ourselves in a positive frame of mind and managing our emotions and stress levels can involve good self-care routines, such as deep breathing, meditation, regular exercise, adequate sleep, nutritional eating, and sharing with a friend. How we deal with excess stress and anxiety can be challenging, but reducing pharmaceutical use as our first go-to method of coping also helps reduce the risk of excess medications inadvertently polluting the water. Return unused OTC or prescriptions drugs to pharmacies. When we are in emotional and mental balance, we will make better choices. We can remain more conscious in how we view and treat the earth and take the time to learn how to reuse, recycle, and dispose of our goods. [21]

Food: We have already looked at aspects of our nutrition, diets, and food consumption and its relationship to financial income. Being able to financially afford to eat healthier foods, pesticide-free vegetables, organic fruit and proteins, as examples, can be challenging for many people. If possible, learn to grow your own food to obtain more nutritional benefits and create a better atmosphere. Eating whole foods more often is a long-term investment into our physical health, and combined with practices that also support good mental health, like eating less sugar substances, can lend itself to healthier lifestyles, potentially fewer physician visits, and lower health costs.

Water: We can use less water and reduce more runoff into our lakes, streams, and oceans. We can take better care of water by not using harmful chemicals in our homes that end up flowing out into our water systems. We can stop using plastic bottled water and invest in filtered water systems instead.

Plastics: If we purchase and store our food in non-plastic bags and containers, it will help reduce plastics use; with the plastics now degrading, micro-plastics are being discovered flowing through our food, in our water, and eventually into our bodies. Choose to reduce, recycle, and then eventually replace plastics with glass, paper, cloth, or reusable biodegradable materials. Composting as much as possible is absolutely essential.

---

[21] For more information on resources for assisting in earth's health and recovery, including tree planting organizations, see appendix D.

Ultimate Self-Care

Clothing: Avoid synthetics as much as possible; chemical processes in some clothes can leach onto your skin and into the water when washing. Bearing in mind that our skin is our largest body organ, adding a form of pollutant next to your skin can cause irritations at minimum and, if left discarded, can also add to more earth pollutants. Search for other whole, organic materials now coming into the market such as, bamboo, hemp, ramie, lyocell, or organic cotton and linen as preferable materials.

A good idea is to go through all the rooms in your home, perhaps beginning with the bathroom and ending in your kitchen, and check to see if there are any items that can be recycled, reused, or replaced with environmentally safer products. This will take your own research, time, and attention. But if we truly want to be supportive to our earth and not just pay lip service while we watch our planet's deterioration, we must all do our part to learn what we can do to help. Just as a simple start, find a good place to plant a tree.

Send Healing Thoughts to Earth

One of the many things we can do for our planet, besides being mindful of integrating as many green environmental strategies as possible, is to send our positive thoughts of love and healing to the earth. As I mentioned in an earlier chapter, we know that thoughts of love and gratitude have a very positive energetic impact on humans, animals, and plants.

For example, in any given moment, when I walk by the ocean or some other waterway, I try to remember to send the water thoughts of love and gratitude. I just say, "I bless the waters with love and gratitude." I send similar thoughts when I walk near a forest, or by rock places, or any area that has earth's growth. I practice sending love and healing to this entire planet and to all the animals and plant life.

We can also visualize the waters and the air being clean and pure and earth's life being restored. Visualizing how we want our planet to look in wellness will aid in the balancing and restorative processes.

Our Way through with Love

> *The greatest power that a human possesses is the power of pure love.*
> —Debasish Mridha

We seem to be in the process of spiritually shifting, of waking up and opening our hearts and minds to the reality that we can eventually transcend to a more loving race of beings, which we actually are at our core. I say this as I am experiencing an acceleration of internet programs, forums, spiritual groups, podcasts, speakers, books, energy/intuitive readers, and love-based mind, body, spirit practitioners. Even some politicians are promoting their awareness of our ability to create more loving, peaceful, and healthy lives within our own communities and in connection to all of earth.

This awareness as we connect with like-minded souls across international communities to promote heart-mind transformations, is a way that humanity can both join with our living earth and work cooperatively, to move away from archaic, disempowering systems that exploit earth's

Ultimate Self-Care

resources, to one where we govern our lives by embracing the powerful attributes of love, peace, and respect for the sacredness of all life. Our way through the chaos and stress is by embracing love.

We will also need to be vigilant in all the practical issues wherever we are on this planet, to ensure we are as prepared as possible to get through the earth's dramatic shifts and extreme climate changes. There will be the obvious need to be knowledgeable in all of our living preparations, in taking stock of essential survival needs in terms of finances, nutrition, medical services, housing, and connecting with others through a sense of community and friendship.

We can still go forward where we are and use our energies wisely for ourselves, in our work, and in the care of our families and community. We can continue to stand up for earth's creature kingdoms that need our help to survive in the water, on land, and in the sky. We can still embrace our creative gifts, skills, and talents, and listen to our heart's yearnings to follow and co-create a joyful path.

Emotionally and spiritually, the attributes of love, such as empathy, compassion, and forgiveness, are some of the key conscious practices that have carried me on my life's journey, kept me safe, and brought me healing and more happiness. These are also the mindful spiritual and emotional states I focus on if I am thrown off course from any sudden change or difficult situation. The energy of love is ultimately a stabilizing force; love acts as an anchor. It transcends time and circumstance.

Practicing nourishing self-care ultimately becomes a powerful way to show the love for ourselves that we deserve. I would venture to say that it is really a lifelong learning for many of us (and it certainly has been for me), an expression of a deeper need to love, cherish, and even heal ourselves. It is a journey that can begin with simple thoughts, such as, *I care about myself; I am worthy to receive all that I need; I am enough as I am; I love myself.*

In time, strengthening the ways we care for and build trust in ourselves will lead us to more confidence and inner peace. With our ability to learn to love and honor who we truly are, when we can awaken the love at the core of our being, we can go forward in our lives, being more fully awake and more consciously aware.

We do need to be prepared, aware, and resourceful to carry us through the range and magnitude of the challenges that are being posed by all the environmental changes and rapid shifts in global systems under way.

As we choose to intentionally express our inherent loving natures, we will continue to open to our greatest source of strength: the wisdom of our hearts, our spirits, and our creative minds. In this way, we can fully manifest problem-solving skills needed for all manner of challenges that arise.

We are all in this together, as it is meant to be. No matter who or where we are, we essentially seek the same things: to feel safe, to feel worthy, to be loved and cared about, to have a sense of belonging, to feel we can participate in a meaningful way as we live our lives, to express our creativity, and to feel genuine happiness.

We can easily see in these times how we are all energetically connected and part of the larger global family. That means that each one of us already plays a vital role in helping to increase the loving consciousness presently

Ultimate Self-Care

unfolding on this planet. We do this by recognizing the sacredness of our own lives and choosing ways to become more nourishing and loving toward ourselves. Beginning with simple, positive self-care steps, we can move toward not only improving the quality of our own lives, but also positively influencing the energy of those around us, including the plants and animals we care for, and even the energy of the earth itself.

CHAPTER 9

CONCLUSION

Self-care will take you further.

We have covered a lot of ground in these pages. What I want to emphasize through everything that has been presented to you is this: Self-care will absolutely empower you. It will make you stronger in every way possible. It will lift up the energies of other people by what they see, sense, and feel in how you respectfully, mindfully, and lovingly strive to honor your own energy, your own needs.

Practicing good self-care also inspires compassion and self-acceptance for who we all are, exactly as we are. When we embrace a loving, compassionate view of ourselves in listening and attending to our nourishment, we can no longer judge ourselves harshly. While no person and no situation is perfect, nurturing ourselves more with supportive practices eventually carries us past the perfectionist demands many of us grew up with. We become a gentler people, a more loving society.

As does anything that really matters to us, caring for ourselves requires a measure of focus, effort, and discipline, but each of us is worth it. We are worth our own investment, attention, and time. I know from my own experiences that taking even one small step toward supporting my own health first has an immediate positive psychological impact.

Barbara Halcrow, MSW

I instantly feel good about myself in what I am doing, and it spurs me on.

You are worth getting to know: how you truly feel, what really matters to you, what fuels your passions, opens your heart, and speaks to the highest visions for yourself. Giving yourself permission to fully nourish yourself as much as you can, and know you deserve it, will magnetize the kind of life you want.

As I write this conclusion, I am reminded that throughout my life, I have felt more in tune with myself, in what I need to do and how I am being guided on my journey, when I am feeling heart-centered. If you are not clear on how to begin any area of your self-care, you may want to start with my own practice by addressing your inner spirit.

I begin my day with gratitude for all I have, all the forms of abundance, for the learning and directions I am given in various ways. As I awaken and just before getting up, I take the initial step of giving gratitude, giving thanks to the loving energy that surrounds me, for all my abundance, for my family and friends, for my work; I thank those who have already passed on to spirit world for their love. I thank spirit for lovingly guiding me.

This expression of gratitude sets the tone of the day. It connects me to the energy of my heart. I then feel more connected to my intuition. Next, I visualize how I want my day to unfold, what I want it to look like in a positive way in anything I want or need to do. Lastly, I look toward the end of the day and imagine how I want to see myself positively feeling. This is exactly how I begin my own self-care, my self-nourishing practice. It works very well for me.

Ultimate Self-Care

Almost on a daily basis, I also try to remember to step back and view events from a larger perspective. At this particular time in our lives, the stakes are very high for the future of humanity and for our earth. I believe, though, that we are actually witnessing a shift in global consciousness toward the need for more feminine energy on the planet, energy that is loving, life-affirming, and contained in the core of us all. I sense this global shift, and it will likely continue to gain strength in all our systems, as we move away from oppressive imbalances that have manifested in economic corruption, oppression, wars, poverty, and illness.

I must emphasize that each of us plays a vital role in this change of consciousness. We are all part of this larger life-affirming, transformative healing process, even if we are not fully aware of it. Remembering we are beings of energy, we can use our individual energy to get more in tune with ourselves, with one another, and with our planet. We do this naturally through more self-nourishment and reflection. As our thoughts move more to the positive, we create an energetic rippling affect that continues to spread throughout our human consciousness.

Seeing ourselves as part of the human collective, a rich, diverse family, we can join together in more ways that can have tremendous positive power to turn all things around as we act in loving cohesiveness. I believe we have already begun, and earth's severe climate changes appear catalystic in bringing many of us closer together in kindness and caring to survive these calamities.

It is understandable to feel overwhelmed with all that is occurring with our earth's changes, with the devastating superstorms occurring more frequently. As I write this, the

Barbara Halcrow, MSW

Amazon is still burning and Hurricane Dorian has left enormous devastation and loss of life in its wake. I realize there is more to come, and we will all be affected in varying ways.

However, in all of this and in your daily routines, there are solutions available to all challenges, especially when we are able to de-stress and take the time to open our hearts and minds and listen to any of the signs and messages that come to us. We are all connected to the divine, to the great intelligence of our universe. We only need to ask for the help we need and then take action when we feel prompted.

Our individual and collective health and wellness, and that of the earth, begins with each one of us. We can start with simple steps in how we can show ourselves the respect, love, and care we deserve.

Wherever you are, I hope that in your life's journey, you will appreciate how your own courage, strength of spirit, and inner beauty have brought you here. May the power of love lead you on.

BIBLIOGRAPHY

American Psychological Association. *The Road to Resilience.* http://www.apa.org/helpcenter/road-resilience.aspx, 2016.

Baker, C. *Collapsing Consciously: Transformative Truths for Turbulent Times.* Berkley, California: North Atlantic Books, 2013.

Barrett, S. *Secrets of Your Cells: Discovering Your Body's Inner Intelligence.* Boulder, CO: Sounds True Inc., 2013.

Bartlett, R. *Matrix Energetics.* New York: Atria Paperback, 2007.

Bayliss, C.R., N. L. Bishop, and RC Fowler, "Pineal Gland Calcification and the Defective Sense of Direction." *British Medical Journal* 291, 21–28, December 1985. (https://www.ncbi.nlm.nih.gov/pmc/articles/PMC1419179/)

Beaudoin, Luc. mysleepapp.com. Global News. http://globalnews.ca/news/3423143/b-c-professors-sleep-technique-gets-attention-from-oprah/, 2017.

Berry, Thomas. *The Dream of the Earth.* San Francisco: Sierra Club Books, 1988.

Bittman, Dr. Barry. "Group Drumming and Neuroendocrine-Immune Parameters," *Alternative Therapies*, 7, no. 1, 38–47, http://drumsofhumanity.org/wpcontent/uploads/2012/01/Immune-System-Study.pdf January 2001.

Black, Jan, and Greg Enns. *Better Boundaries. Owning and Treasuring Your Life.* Oakland, CA: New Harbinger Publishers, 1997.

Blum, Ralph. *The Book of Runes.* New York: Oracle Books, St. Martin's Press, 1987.

Braden, Gregg. *Resilience from the Heart. The Power to Thrive in Life's Extremes.* Hay House Publishers, 2015.

Bridges, William. *Managing Transitions: Making the Most of Change.* Philadelphia: William Bridges and Associates, Perseus Books Group, 2009.

Burney, Diana. *Spiritual Clearings: Sacred Practices to Release Negative Energy and Harmonize Your life.* Berkeley, CA: North Atlantic Books, 2009.

Canada Safety Council. Canadasafetycouncil.org https://canadasafetycouncil.org/safety-canadaonline/article/driver-fatigue-falling-asleep-wheel.online/issue/vol-liii-no-2-april-2009.

Canadian Sleep Review, *Current Issues, Attitudes, and Advice to Canadians.* Developed in consultation with the Canadian Sleep Review Panel with support from Dairy Farmers of Canada. May 2016.

Chakra-Anatomy.com. https://www.chakra-anatomy.com, 2016.

Chambers, Dr. Lin. "What Wavelength Goes with What Colour?" www.science-edu.larc.nasa.gov, 2016.

Chiasson, Ann Marie. *Energy Healing: The Essentials of Self-Care.* Boulder, CO: Sounds True, Inc., 2013.

Cichoke, Anthony J. *Secrets of Native American Herbal Remedies: A Comprehensive Guide to the Native American Tradition of Using Herbs and the Mind/Body/Spirit Connection for Improving Health and Well-Being.* New York: Penguin Publishers, 2001.

Chopra, Deepak, and Rudolph E. Tanzi. *Super Brain: Unleashing the Explosive Power of Your Mind to Maximize Health, Happiness, and Spiritual Well-Being.* New York: Harmony Books, 2012.

Chopra, Deepak. *Ageless Body, Timeless Mind: The Quantum Alternative to Growing Old.* New York: Three Rivers Press, 2010.

Collins New English Dictionary. Great Britain: HarperCollins Publishers, 1998.

Coon, Robert. *Earth Chakras: The Definitive Guide.* Raleigh, North Carolina: Lulu Press, 2009.

Coon, Robert, http://earthchakras.org/Books.php

Coon, Robert, http://earthchakras.org/Locations.php

Cooper, Diana. *Angel Answers*. Scotland, UK: Findhorn Press, 2007.

Dangeli, Jevon. *Bio-Communication*. 2007–2017, https://jevondangeli.com/bio-communication/

Doidge, Norman. *The Brain That Changes Itself: Stories of Personal Triumph from the Frontiers of Brain Science.* New York: Penguin Books, 2007.

Duck, J. D. *Managing the Change: The Art of Balancing,* https://hbr.org/1993/11/managing-change-the-art-of-balancing, November-December Issue, 1993. par. 24), 1993.

Dyer, W. *Change Your Thoughts, Change Your Life*. Hay House Publishing, 2007.

Emoto, Masaru. *The Hidden Messages in Water*. New York: Atria Books, 2009.

First Nations Traditional Foods Fact Sheets. First Nations Health Authority: fnha.ca, 2016, http://www.fnha.ca/wellnessContent/Wellness/Traditional Food Facts Sheets.pdf

Fosar, Grazyna, and Franz Bludorf. "Scientists Prove DNA Can Be Reprogrammed by Words and Frequencies," originally taken from the book *Vernetzie Intelligenz,* http://wakeup-world.com/2011/07/12/scientistprove-dna-can-be-reprogrammed-by-words-frequencies/

Frost, Robert. "Mending Wall," in *North of Boston*. David Nutt. 1914.

Gagliano, Monica. *The Science of Plant Behaviour and Consciousness,* http://www.monicagagliano.com.

Gawain, Shakti. *Creative Visualization*. New Delhi, India: Nataraj Publishing, 2002.

Geiger, John. *The Angel Effect*. New York: Weinstein Books, 2013.

Gerber, Richard. *Vibrational Medicine. The #1 Handbook of Subtle-Energy Therapies,* Third Edition. Rochester, Vermont: Bear & Co., 2001.

Graham, Linda. *Bouncing Back: Rewiring Your Brain for Maximum Resilience and Well-Being*. Novato, CA: New World Library, 2013.

Goodreads. A Nutritional Reading List, https://www.goodreads.com/list/show/7183.A_Nutrition_Reading_List

Hall, Judith. *The Crystal Bible*. Great Britain: Godsfield Press, 2003.

Halpern, Steven. *Chakra Suite*. Halpern Inner Peace Music. www.StevenHalpern.com.

Hawkins, David R. *Power vs Force: The Hidden Determinant of Human Behavior*. Hay House, CA, 2012.

Hay, Louise. *You Can Heal Your Life*. Hay House Inc., 1984.

Hay, Louise. *Life!* Hay House Publishers, 1996.

Hensrud, D. "Is Too Little Sleep a Cause of Weight Gain?" In *Sleep and Weight Gain: What's the Connection?* https://www.mayoclinic.org/healthy-lifestyle/adult-health/expert-answers/sleep-and-weight-gain/faq-20058198, 2015.

Hicks, Esther, and Jerry. *Ask and It Is Given. Learning to Manifest Your Desires*. Carlsbad, CA, New Delhi: Hay House, Inc., 2004.

Hoberman Levine, Barbara. *Your Body Believes Every Word You Say*. Santa Rosa, CA: Aslan Publishing, 1991.

Indigenous Performing Arts Alliance. "Smudging Document, Smudging and Protocol Guidelines" (www.cda-acd./docs/advocacy/smudging-Document-June-2015.pdf).

Institute of Noetic Sciences. *Defining Noetic Sciences*. https://noetic.org/about/origins/

Jampolsky, Gerald C. *Forgiveness: The Greatest Healer of All*. New York: Atira Paperback; Hillsboro, Oregon: Beyond Words, 2007.

Johns Hopkins Medicine. *3 Kinds of Exercises That Boost Heart Health*. The Johns Hopkins University, the Johns Hopkins Health System, https://www.hopkinsmedicine.org/health/wellness-and-prevention/3-kinds-of-exercise-that-boost-heart-health

Johnson, David. *Do Different Colours Affect Your Mood? Colours, Meanings and Moods.* Colour Psychology 2000-2016, http://www.infoplease.com/spot/colors1.html

Kuthumi quote, from Milanovich, Dr. Norma, and Dr. Shirley McCune. *The Light Shall Set You Free,* 4th Edition. 1996. Kalispell, Montana: Athena Publishing.

Levitin, Daniel, and Mona Lisa Chandra. "Trends in Cognitive Science." *The Neurochemistry of Music Journal,* Department of Psychology, McGill University, Montreal, Quebec, QC H3A 1B1, Canada https://daniellevitin.com/levitinlab/articles/2013-TICS_1180.pdf

Linden, Anne. *Boundaries in Human Relationships: How to Be Separated and Connected.* Crown House Publishing Ltd. and Crown House Publishing Company LLC., CT http://www.goodreads.com/quotes/tag/boundaries, 2008

Lipton, Bruce H. *The Biology of Belief. Unleashing the Power of Consciousness, Matter and Miracles.* Hay House, 2015.

Lewis, C. S. *The Four Loves.* London: Cox & Wyman Ltd., Fakenham, for the publishers Geoffrey Bles Ltd., 1960.

Lindenfield, G. *Assertive Bill of Rights.* United Kingdom (http://www.gaellindenfield.com), 2016

Lousma, Jack. "Preface" in *Pathways of Understanding: The Interactions of Humanity and Global Environmental Change* (https://www.ciesin.columbia.edu/documents/CIESIN1992PathwaysofUnderstanding_sm.pdf), University Centre,

Michigan: Centre for International Earth Science Information Network, 1992.

Luke, Jennifer. School of Biological Sciences, University of Surrey, Guilford, UK, Department of Obstetrics and Gynaecology, The Royal London Hospital, abstract, "Fluoride Deposition in the Human Pineal Gland," in the International Center for Nutritional Research, 2001 (http://www.icnr.com/articles/fluoride-deposition.html).

Ma'ati Smith, Dr. Jane. *Chakra Healing Sounds,* http://balance.chakrahealingsounds.com/the-7-chakras

MacLean, Kenneth, and Michael James. *The Vibrational Universe: Harnessing the Power of Thought to Consciously Create Your Life.* Baker and Taylor, Ingram Book Group, New Leaf Distributing, Loving Healing Press, 2006.

Manning, B., and R. Bennett. *Abba's Child: The Cry of the Heart for Intimate Belonging.* NavPress Publishing Group (http://www.goodreads.com/work/quotes/513762), 2002.

Markowitz, D. *Self-Care for the Self-Aware. A Guide for Highly Sensitive People, Empaths, Intuitives, and Healers.* Bloomington, Indiana: Balboa Press, 2013.

Martinex-Conde, Susana, and Stephen L. Machknik. "How the Colour Red Influences Our Behaviour." *Scientific America, Behaviour and Society* 01.11, 2014.

Mate, Gabor. *When the Body Says No: The Cost of Hidden Stress.* Vintage Canada, a division of Random House, 2012.

Mathieu, F. *Running on Empty: Compassion Fatigue in Health Professionals,* http://www.compassionfatigue.org/pages/RunningOnEmpty.pdf, 2007

Mathieu, F. "Compassion Fatigue: What You Don't Know Will Hurt You." This Changed My Practice (UBC, CPD), University of British Columbia, https://www.google.ca/search?safe=active&q=http://this+changed+my+practice/com/compassion-

McNally, Jess. "Earth's Most Stunning Natural Fractal Patterns." *Science*. 09.10.10. https://www.wired.com/author/j_mcnally

McNeil, Barbara. 2006. "Cosmic Activist" (online article) in *Shift: At the Frontiers of Consciousness*, no. 12, September–November 2006, https://noetic.org/about/noetic-sciences/

Meditation Freedom: Chakra Balancing and Healing Meditation Music with Crystal Bowls, https://www.youtube.com/

Melchizedek, Drunvalo. *The Ancient Secret of the Flower of Life.* Flagstaff, Arizona: Clear Light Trust, Light Technology Publishing, 1998.

Milanovich, Dr. Norma J., and Dr. Shirley McCune. *The Light Shall Set You Free,* 4th Edition. Kalispell, Montana: Athena Publishing, 1996.

Millman, Dan. *Way of the Peaceful Warrior.* Tiburon, California: New World Library, 2002.

Mindell, Earl. *Earl Mindell's New Herb Bible.* New York: Fireside, Simon & Schuster, 2000.

Mridha, D. quote from Goodreads, http://www.goodreads.com/author/show/7441013

Moerman, Daniel. *Native American Ethnobotany.* Timber Press, http://www.herbmed.org/links.html, 1998.

Moskowitz, Clara. "Fact or Fiction? Energy Can Neither Be Created nor Destroyed." *Scientific American.* Aug. 5, 2014.

Murakami, Haruki. *Norwegian Wood.* Vintage International Original, 2000.

Myss, Carolyn. *Anatomy of the Spirit.* New York: Harmony Books, Random House, 1996.

National Research Council, Division on Earth and Life Studies, Board on Environmental Studies and Toxicology, Committee on Fluoride in Drinking Water. *Fluoride in Drinking Water: A Scientific Review of EPA Standards.* National Academic Press. Jan. 22, 2007, 256, https://www.google.ca/search?tbo=p&tbm=bks&q=inauthor:%22Division+on+Earth+and+Life+Studies%22

National Institute of General Medical Sciences. *Circadian Rhythm Fact Sheet,* 04.06.2016, https://www.nigms.nih.gov/Education/Pages/Factsheet_CircadianRhythms.asp

Paris Agreement. *Paris Agreement/Climate Action,* https://unfccc.int/process-and-meetings/the-paris-agreement/the-paris-agreement

Pearce, Eiluned, and Jacques Launay. "The Ice-Breaker Effect: Singing Mediates Fast Social Bonding." *Royal Society Open Science,* October: doi: 10.1098/rsos.150221.

Pert, Candice. *Molecules of Emotion: The Science behind Mind-Body Medicine.* New York: Scribner Publishers, 1997.

Pert, Candice. *Where Do You Store Your Emotions?* The Institute of Medicine, 2008–2016, http://candacepert.com/where-do-you-store-youremotions/

Povah, L. *Drum Circle Program for Eating Disorders.* Saint Paul's Hospital, Vancouver, BC, http://drummingandhealth.com/wpcontent/uploads/2012/07/Research-Study-Results-DrumCircle-Program-2011.pdf, 2011.

Price, J. R. *The Superbeings. The Superselling Guide to Finding Your Higher Self.* New York: Fawcett Books, 1987.

Priest, S., and M. Gass. "An Examination of 'Problem-Solving' versus 'Solution-Focused' in a Corporate Setting." In *Association for Experimental Education* 20, no. 1, May 1997 34–37, https://journals.sagepub.com/doi/10.1177/105382599702000106

Prophet, E. C. *The Violet Flame to Heal Body, Mind and Soul.* Gardiner, Montana: Summit University Press, 1997.

Public Health Agency of Canada. "Population Health. What Determines Health? Key Determinants." http://www.phac-aspc.gc.ca/ph-sp/determinants/indexeng.php#key_determinants

Ray, A. *Mindfulness: Living in the Moment, Living in the Breath.* Inner Light Publishers, 2015.

Rendel, P. *Understanding Chakras: Discovering and Using the Energy of Your Seven Vital Force Centres.* Wellingborough, North Hamptonshire, England: Aquarian Press, Thorsons Publishing Group, 1990.

Reuben, Mischa. "The Earth's Next 100 Years, Visualized." *Upworthy,* Dec. 11, 2013, www.upworthy.com/the-future-of-the-earth-s-next-100years-visualized

Ritchie, George G. *Return from Tomorrow.* Grand Rapids, MI: Flemming H. Revel, Baker Book House, 1978.

Rome, D. I. *Your Body Knows the Answer: Using Your Felt Sense to Solve Problems, Affect Change, and Liberate Creativity.* Boston: Shambhala Publications, Inc., 2014.

Shiv, Vandana. *Golden Rice: Myth, Not Miracle.* 2014 (http://gmwatch.org/index.php/news/archive/2014/15250golden-rice-myth-not-miracle).

Siegal, B. "Love: The Healer," in Carlson, Richard, and Benjamin Shield, Eds. *Healers on Healing.* Los Angeles: St. Martin's Press, 1989.

Silver Birch Series. *Teachings of Silver Birch.* Edited by Austen, A.W. Spiritual Truth Foundation, Booksprint Printers, GB, 1998.

Skinner, S. *Sacred Geometry: Deciphering the Code.* New York: Sterling Publishing Co., 2006.

"Smudging Ceremony, Native American Customs & Traditions" (https://powwow-power.com/smudging/).

Speers, P., and T. Walker. *The Inspired Caregiver: Finding Joy while Caring for Those You Love.* Monterey, CA: Flowspirations, 2013.

Sun Bear with Wabun Wind. *Black Dawn Bright Day: Indian Prophecies for the Millennium that Reveal the Fate of the Earth.*, New York: Fireside, Simon and Schuster, 1992.

The Australian. Editorial: "Europe's Compassion Fatigue." September 17, 2015, theAustralian.com.au, http://www.theaustralian.com.au/opinion/editorials/europes-compassion-fatigue/

The Harvard Medical School. "5 of the Best Exercises You Can Ever Do." *Healthbeat*. Harvard Medical School. Harvard Health Publishing. 2016–2019, https://www.health.harvard.edu/staying-healthy/5-of-the-best-exercises-you-can-ever-do

The Self Help Alliance, University of Alberta. "Building Better Boundaries." https://cloudfront.ualberta.ca/-/media/medicine/departments/anesthesiology/documents/workbookbuilding-better-boundariesfeb2011.pdf

Tucker, Dr. Jim, and Ian Stevenson. *Life before Life: A Scientific Investigation of Children's Memories of Previous Lives*. New York: St. Martin's Griffin, 2008.

Turtle Island Native Network: "Healing and Wellness," http://www.turtleisland.org/healing/healing-wellness.htm

Vaag, Jonas, Per Øystein Saksvik, Töres Theorell, Trond Skillingstad, and, Ottar Bjerkeset. "The Sound of Well-Being: Choir Singing as an Intervention to Improve Well-Being among Employees in Two Norwegian County Hospitals," in *Science Nordic*, Nov. 12. 2012.

Violet Flame. *The Secret of the Violet Flame*. http://violetflame.com/violet-flame-secret/, 2016.

Virtual Sports Injury Clinic. https://www.sportsinjuryclinic.net

Virtue, D., and J. Lukomski. *Crystal Therapy: How to Heal and Empower Your Life with Crystal Energy*. Hay House, 2005.

Virtue, D. *Chakra Clearing: Awakening Your Spiritual Power to Know and Heal*. Hay House, Inc., 1998.

Virtue, D. *Healing with the Angels*. Hay House Inc., 1999.

Virtue, D. *Angel Numbers, 101. The Meaning of 111, 123, 444, and Other Number Sequences*. Hay House, 2008.

Wang, Christine. "Symbolism of Color and Color Meanings around the World." www.shutterstock.com/blog/color-symbolism-andmeanings-around-the-world, 2008.

Watson, Brenda. *The DETOX Strategy, Vibrant Health in 5 Easy Steps*. New York: Free Press, 2008.

Weil, Andrew. *Spontaneous Healing*. New York: Ballantine Publishing Co., 1995.

Weil, A. "Dr. Weil's Breathing Exercises: 4-7-8." http://www.drweil.com/videos-features/videos/the-4-7-8breath-health-benefits-demonstration/

Wikipedia. Pineal Gland (https://en.wikipedia.org/wiki/Pineal_gland).

Wilde, Stuart. *Affirmations*. Taos, New Mexico: Dove International Inc., 1987.

Wilde, Stuart. *The Quickening*. Hay House Inc., 1988.

Wills, Pauline. "Colour Therapy," in *Health Essentials: The Use of Colour for Health and Healing*. Great Britain: Element Books, 1993.

Wolfe, David "Avocado,." Living Nutrition e-course, the BodyMind Institute, https://shop.davidwolfe.com/products/david-avocado-wolfe-living-nutrition-e-course

Wright, Angela. *The Colour Affect Systems. Colour Affects.* https://www.researchgate.net/publication/253271089_The_Colour_Affects_System_of_Colour_Psychology, 2008-2016

APPENDIX A

RESOURCES FOR FURTHER INTUITIVE DEVELOPMENT

There are many informal and formal ways to develop our additional senses. There are credible institutes that offer formal trainings, such as the Arthur Findlay College in Stansted, England, which I had opportunity to attend. There are many other settings locally and worldwide, that offer a range of structured retreats and inner journeying with excellent teachers. One can also search for local trusted spiritual community groups to bring forward one's spiritual development and expression in a manner that feels right. Here are some other resources:

Hollyhock, BC: https://hollyhock.ca/experience

Chopra Center Personal Growth Retreats: https://chopra.com/personal-and-spiritual-growth

Depending on the environment and experience one is looking for, life-enhancing retreats are located throughout the world. Besides checking with a resource person in your community, the website below may steer you in the right direction and offer some ideas:

https://www.bookmeditationretreats.com/all/c/spiritual-retreats

There are also many things we can do easily on a daily basis through personal meditations, creativity or artwork, music, play, and spending time with animals or being out in our natural surroundings. All of these and more will stimulate and enhance your spiritual senses.

APPENDIX B

RESOURCES FOR GUIDED MEDITATIONS

The following websites may interest those who want to download guided meditations and subliminal recordings:

The Chopra Center: Guided Meditations: https://chopra.com/articles/guided-meditations

Hay House Personal Meditations for Healing: https://www.hayhouse.com/meditations-for-personal-healing-1

Kelly Howells's Brain Sync website has numerous excellent quality offerings for purchase and one free guided download: https://www.brainsync.com/free-guided-meditation-online

Conscious Panda: The 10 Best Guided Meditation Sites: https://consciouspanda.com/best-guided-meditation-sites/

Hero Movement: Twelve of the Best Free Guided Meditation Sites in 2018: https://www.heromovement.net/blog/free-guided-meditation-resources/

APPENDIX C

RESOURCES FOR COCREATING, AFFIRMING, AND MANIFESTING

Dyer, Wayne. *Change Your Thoughts, Change Your Life.* Hay House Publishing, 2007.

Gawain, Shakti. *Creative Visualization.* Nataraj Publishing; Division of New World Library, 2002.

Hay, Louise. *You Can Heal Your Life.* Hay House Publishers, 1984.

Hay, Louise. *Life!* Hay House Publishers, 1996.

Hicks, Esther, and Jerry. *Ask and It Is Given.* Hay House Publishing, 2004.

Wilde, Stuart. *Affirmations.* Taos, New Mexico: Dove International Inc., 1987.

Wilde, Stuart. *The Quickening.* Hay House Inc., 1988.

Goodreads: Most Popular Manifesting books: https://www.goodreads.com/shelf/show/manifesting

You Tube has an array of videos on manifesting, guided meditations, and affirmations.

APPENDIX D

RESOURCES TO ASSIST IN EARTH'S HEALTH

David Suzuki Foundation: https://www.davidsuzuki.org

Green America: https://www.greenamerica.org/green-living/10-habits-highly-sustainable

Go Green Initiative: https://gogreeninitiative.org

Top 100 Sites for Going Green: https://www.environmentalsciencedegree.com/green-living/

Tree Planting Websites

WeForest: https://www.weforest.org

Replant.ca: http://www.replant.ca/index.html

The Nature Conservatory: https://www.nature.org/en-us/get-involved/how-to-help/plant-a-billion/

APPENDIX E

SUGGESTIONS FOR BUILDING A SELF-CARE PLAN

Step 1: Self-Care Assessment

A self-care assessment is a nonjudgmental self-assessment of personal strengths and vulnerabilities in how we structure and balance our daily activities, in addition to our strategies in coping with stress.

Consider the categories of mind, body, emotion, and spirit and ask yourself these questions:

- In what ways do I already actively support my mental, physical, emotional, and spiritual needs?
- What areas need more support, and do I have plans to meet them?
- Do I have enough of a work/home balance?
- How do I cope with stress, positively or negatively?
- Are there short-term changes I can make to improve my self-care plan?
- What kind of assistance do I need to make other necessary changes to my self-care plan?

Self-Care Assessment Checklist

Tick off the areas you already participate in then and highlight other areas you want to initiate:

Physical

- Sufficient sleep
- Healthy eating
- Hydration
- Daily exercise
- Relaxation time-outs during the day
- Time alone during the day
- Time out in nature
- Deep breathing
- Listen to your body to find areas of stress
- Massage or other complimentary relaxation methods
- Short or longer-term vacations
- Other:

Psychological

- Reading for interest/enjoyment
- Forms of puzzles for mind exercises
- Games with yourself or others
- Personal writing (journaling)
- Deep breathing or meditation for mind calming
- Spend time in nature
- Short- or long-term vacations

- Lighten yourself with activities that promote laughter
- Attend new events and share ideas with different people
- Practice not analyzing situations or people
- Turn off the news
- Decide to learn something new and fun
- See where you are naturally creative and develop it further
- Know what your boundaries are and respect them
- Other:

Emotional

- Connect with people you've not seen for a while
- Spend time with positive people who support your best interests
- Look for your own strengths and accomplishments and congratulate yourself by word and deeds
- Tell yourself as much as you can, "I love you."
- Listen to good music, attend a play, or go to a concert
- Sing or join a choir for your own enjoyment
- Dine in an expensive restaurant because you deserve it
- See a support person to deal with anxieties, traumas, or addictions
- Volunteer where it is not overly stressful
- Regulate or turn off the news
- Other:

Spiritual

- Deep breathing and forms of meditation
- Walk in nature and breathe in the life force all around you
- Spend time with animals
- Spend time with plants or in a garden
- Go inside your heart and ask how it feels or what it wants to do
- Read or listen to something daily that inspires you
- Repeat statements daily that affirm your strengths, your deepest wishes for how you want to see your life unfold
- Think of what you are grateful for
- Forgive and accept yourself and others as much as possible
- Practice random acts of kindness
- Spend time in a spiritual group that uplifts you
- Practice allowing things to flow (letting go of needing to control)
- Allow others to give to you
- Tell people something you like or appreciate about them
- Appreciate the journey of courage you are on

Step 2: Daily and Weekly Planning

Daily and weekly routines may work for others but not for you. Implement the easiest, smaller strategies first.

- Maintain already established healthy areas.

- Add in self-care practices in more vulnerable areas.
- Structure in a daily and then weekly routine.

Step 3: Commitment and Follow-Through

- Make a commitment on a daily basis to follow-through on your plan.
- Make adjustments as necessary.

Step 4: Structure in Support for Commitment

- Always plan self-care routines a day ahead.
- Prepare for challenges or emergency situations.
- Structure in visible or technical reminders.
- Share your plan with others.
- Participate in similar activities with others.
- Keep congratulating yourself for any positive changes you make.
- Be gentle and patient with yourself.
- Affirm your well-being.

INDEX

A

Aboriginal, 134
Abydos, 182–83
acupuncture, 20, 60
Aeon Activation, 181
affirmations, 155, 172, 225
akashic records, 11
Effect, The (Geiger), 86, 209
angels, 87, 218
anger, 112, 126, 159
animals, 55, 57, 76, 102, 176–78, 222
apathy, 110–11
Archangel Michael, 87–88
Aron, Elaine, 47
Arthur Findlay College, 221
assertiveness, 96
auras, 5–6, 12
auric fields, 6–7, 11–13, 58, 61, 84
Ayurveda, 128

B

Barrett, S, 205
Barrett, Sondra, 26
Bartlett, R, 205
Bartlett, R., 26, 205
Beddoes, Tyler, 86
Bittman, Barry, 75
Black Dawn, 217
blessing, 137
Bloom, William, 87
Bludorf, Franz, 29
body talk, 28
boundaries, 15, 49, 69, 83, 89–96, 99, 110, 116, 169, 206, 211, 217, 231
Braden, Gregg, 152, 206
breathwork, 20–21
Bridges, William, 115–16, 206
Buddha, 92, 113
Byrne, Lorna, 87

C

caregiving, 48, 96, 122
Cayce, Edgar, 43
chakras, 11–17, 64–67, 76–77, 84–85, 139, 142, 179–82, 207, 212, 216
change, 114–16, 124, 126, 150, 197, 203
children, 2, 89–90
Chopra, Deepak, xiii, 102, 207
clairaudience, 42
claircognizance, 44–45
clairvoyance, 11, 43
clearing, 49, 52, 57, 59–65, 70–72, 84
climate changes, xxii, 197, 203
clothing, 195
cocreation, 165, 167, 173

coincidences, 173, 175
colored light, 22
colors, 9–10, 12, 14, 22, 75–80, 85, 135
communication, 16, 104, 106–8
compassion, 120, 149, 156, 160, 177, 201
compassion fatigue, 120–22
consciousness, 3–4, 21, 52, 65, 110, 184–85, 203
Coon, Robert, 179, 182
Cooper, Dianna, 87
cords, 66–67, 69
courage, 110, 112, 232
creativity, 79
crystals, 22, 65–66

D

Dalai Lama, 51
decluttering, 71
default to the negative, 102, 106, 125
desire, 111, 122
drumming, 74–75
Dyer, Wayne, 2, 225

E

earth, 84, 177–80, 184, 188–92, 197, 203
Egypt, 66, 183
emotions, 110
empathy, 16, 46, 110, 120, 158, 164, 197
empower, 201

energy, 5, 7–8, 10, 18, 56, 114, 130, 143, 158
enlightenment, 113
epigenetics, 24–25
etheric cords, 66
extrasensory perception (ESP), 43

F

family caregivers, 121–22
fear, 103, 106, 108, 111, 164
feelings, 34, 58, 99, 150–51, 164
feminine, 79, 203
First Nations, 61, 74, 129, 135
flower essence, 21
Flower of Life, 182–83
fluoridation, 138
food, 128–31, 135–37, 139, 194
forgiveness, 159, 162
Fosar, Grazyna, 29
Agreements, The (Ruiz), 107
fractals, 185
frequencies, 21, 71, 109
Frost, Robert, 209

G

Gagliano, Monica, 74
Garnes, Dee, 2
Geiger, John, 86, 209
gemstones, 22, 65
genetically modified organisms (GMOs), 130
geometry, 183–85
Gerber, Richard, 18, 209

236

Glastonbury, 180
global, xxii, 190, 203, 211
gossip, 107–8
gratitude, 157, 202
Great Pyramid, 66, 180
grief, 111
grounding, 51, 59, 69
guilt, 110–11

H

happiness, xxv, 26, 124, 173
Haruki Murakami, 154
Hawkins, David, 109, 158
healing sound therapies, 21
heart, 16, 54–56, 151–55, 158, 180, 210
herbs, 61, 133–35
Higher Self, 92, 165, 168
Highly Sensitive Person: How to Thrive When the World Overwhelms You, The (Aron), 46
Hippocrates, 18
Hoberman Levine, Barbara, 24, 210
holistic, xxiii, xxv, xxvii, 6, 186
homeopathy, 21

I

imagination, 171–72, 174
Indigenous peoples, 76, 190
inner child, 99
insomnia, 142–43
Institute of Noetic Sciences (IONS), 3
intention, 61–62, 72, 86
intuition, 4, 11, 38–41, 44, 119, 152, 202

J

Jampolsky, G., 159
journalism, 105
joy, 113

K

Krishna, 113
Kuthumi, 152

L

Lake Titicaca, 180
Launay, Jacques, 73
Levitin, Daniel, 74, 211
LGBTQ2S, 127–28
lifestyle, 133, 140–41, 146, 173
Lindenfield, Gael, 98, 211
Lipton, Bruce, 25
Lousma, Jack, 188, 211
love, 68, 112–13, 156, 162–64

M

MacLean, Kenneth, 1, 212
MacQueen, Meg, 186
magnetize, 202
Mahesh, Maharishi, 52
Managing Transitions: Making the Most of Change (Bridges), 115
manifesting, 170
Markowitz, D., 48
Masaru Emoto, 30

Mate, Gabor, 39
mathematics, 183
matrix energetics, 26, 205
Mayo Clinic, 141
McNeil, Barbara, 4
media, 104–5
meditation, 8, 51–55, 164, 185–86, 232
Melchizedek, Drunvalo, 182–84, 213
Melchizedek, Drunvalo, 213
mental health, 193
Middle East, 180
Millman, Dan, 23
mind, 8, 51–52, 63, 101, 112
Mindell, Earl, 135
mindfulness, 129, 162
Morin, C., 142
Moskowitz, Clara, 2, 214
Mount Kailas, 181
Mount Shasta, 179
Mridha, D., 196
Mt. of Olives, 180
Mt. Sinai, 180
Murgatroyd, 187
music, 64, 74, 90, 158
Myss, Carolyn, 6

N

nature, 35, 79, 175–76, 179, 184
near-death experiences, 3
neutrality, 112
Norwegian Wood (Murakami), 154, 214

nutrition, 128, 130, 137, 140, 194. *See also* food

P

Paris Agreement, 189
past-life experiences, 2
peace, 113, 155–56, 158
Pearce, Eiluned, 73, 215
plastics, 194
Povah, Lyle, 75
Power vs. Force: The Hidden Determinations of Human Behaviour (Hawkins), 109
Price, John Randolph, 63
pride, 112
Priest, S., 125
problem-solving, 198

Q

qi gong, 10

R

Ray, Amit, 101
reduce, 106, 141, 145, 193–94
reflexology, 20
Reiki, 18, 20, 65, 160
relationships, 93, 108, 124, 166
repeating numbers, 174
resilience, 123–26, 147
Return from Tomorrow, 216
Ritchie, George G., 3
Ruiz, Don Miguel, 107
Rumi, 3

S

Sacred Geometry, 217
Saint Germain, 85, 113
savikalpa samadhi, 4
Secrets of Your Cells, 205
self-acceptance, 201
self-confidence, xxii, 13, 78, 119
self-esteem, xxii, 13, 112, 126, 166
seniors, 75
sensitivity, 46–47, 83, 109
Shaftesbury, 180
shame, 110–11
Silver Birch, 168
singing, 72–73
smudging, 61, 71
Socrates, 108
Speers, Peggi, 172
spices, 134–35
spirit, 154, 176, 180
spirituality, 80, 149
Stevenson, Ian, 3
stones, 22, 65. *See also* crystals
, The (Price), 63
Super Brain (Chopra and Tanzi), 131, 207
Swami Vivekanada, 113
synchronicity, 173–74

T

tai chi, 10, 21, 146
Tamura, Michael J., 13
Tanzi, Rudolph E., 102, 131–32, 207
Teachings of Silver Birch, 168, 217
Tesla, Nikola, 1
third eye, 17
Tolle, Eckhart, 163
Tompkins, Ptolemy, 86
Transcendental Meditation, 52
transitions, 116, 142
Tucker, Jim, 3

U

Uluru-Kata Tjuta, 180
universal intelligence, 168, 187
University of Oxford, 73
University of Western Australia, 74

V

vibrational medicine, 18–19, 22
Vibrational Universe, 212
vibrations, 52, 73, 113, 156, 175
violet flame, 85
visualize, 60, 162
voice, 72, 152, 155
vulnerability, 84, 151

W

Wabun Wind, 190, 217
Walker, Tia, 172
Wang, Christine, 77, 218
water, 30–31, 137–38, 177, 193–94
Watson, Brenda, 138
weight gain, 141

Weil, Andrew, 53, 131
willingness, 112
Wills, Pauline, 14, 76–77, 219
wisdom, 23, 25, 32, 38, 153
workspace, 70–71

Y

yin and yang, 17
yoga, 10, 21
Your Body Believes Every Word
    You Say, 210

ABOUT THE AUTHOR

Since childhood, Barbara Halcrow was naturally inspired to support, encourage, and help others, and, it was through a near-fatal accident, that she was redirected to begin her life's work as a Social Worker, trainer, and healer. She received her MSW from the University of Manitoba.

On this healing and teaching path, Barbara traveled to diverse urban and rural communities in British Columbia, Manitoba, and the Yukon territory in Canada, as well as Seoul, Korea. Her work primarily involved the areas of child protection, domestic violence, sexual abuse, mental health and addictions, and most recently, in adult/older adult health care. Barbara held many leadership roles across the health care continuum in acute care, rehabilitation, and community care sectors.

Spiritually, being an intuitive, empathic person, Barbara always felt a strong connection to the beauty and power of nature, the realm of spirit, and the vitality of the loving energy that flows through all of life. Over the years, this deep connection led to further spiritual development and energy studies at home and abroad.

Barbara Halcrow studied at Stansted, England's Arthur Findlay College of Spiritualism and Psychic Sciences. She also trained in several levels of the Melchizedek Method from the Kamadon Academy, Australia, and further received certification in Reiki healing in Vancouver, BC. Barbara has also completed a course in medical intuition from the International College of Medical Intuition, Inc. in British Columbia, Canada.

Barbara believes that by offering ourselves more conscious love and self-nourishment, we will gain in personal strength and resiliency. She also acknowledges that by embracing gratitude, compassion, and forgiveness toward ourselves and others, we will enhance our ability to move forward in our sacred life journeys with increased clarity in our direction and purpose. This clarity can create swifter, positive changes in our lives, and in turn, we can more positively affect the lives of others, as well as the health of our earth.